COMPASSION ENERGY

A HEIDEGGERIAN APPROACH

COMPASSION ENERGY

A HEIDEGGERIAN APPROACH

Dorothy J. Dunn

Bethesda Scientific

London-Washington:

Academica Press

Library of Congress Cataloging-in-Publication Data

Names: Dunn, Dorothy J., 1956- author.
Title: Compassion energy : a Heideggerian approach / Dorothy J. Dunn.
Description: London ; Washington, DC : Academica Press, [2018] |
Includes
bibliographical references.
Identifiers: LCCN 2018054613 | ISBN 9781680534733 (hardcover : alk.
paper)
Subjects: | MESH: Heidegger, Martin, 1889-1976. | Nursing Theory |
Empathy |
Nurses--psychology | Nursing Care--psychology | Qualitative Research
Classification: LCC RT41 | NLM WY 86 | DDC 610.73--dc23
LC record available at https://lccn.loc.gov/2018054613

ABSTRACT

The purpose of this study was to explore what keeps nurses in nursing by examining the impact of the relational experiences between the nurse and her or his patient in the context of the nursing situation. Heideggerian hermeneutic phenomenology grounded the study and was the method used to interpret the registered nurse participants' meaning of their everydayness. The nurses' first hand perspectives elicited implications for nursing practice.

This qualitative research study examined what keeps nurses in nursing. The eight registered nurse participants provided rich descriptive data from which four relational themes emerged: Practicing from Inner Core Beliefs, Understanding the Other from Within, Making a Difference, and Nursing as an Evolving Process.

Heideggerian hermeneutic phenomenology was the philosophy that grounded the study and the method used to interpret the nursing situation. The philosophical concepts of Heidegger's *Being and Time* included authenticity, care, choice, conscience, decision, everydayness, responsibility, and being-there (Dasein) were utilized in the analysis. The hermeneutical interpretative process guided the researcher to synthesize the themes into a constitutive pattern of meaning which the researcher named *Intentional Compassion Energy.*

In intentional caring consciousness, the nurse intentionally knows the nursed as whole. Compassion energy is the intersubjective gift of compassion that gives nurses the opportunity to be with the nursed. Compassion energy is composed of compassionate presence, patterned nurturance and intentionally knowing the nursed and self as whole. Thus, intentional compassion energy is defined as the regeneration of nurses' capacity to foster interconnectedness when the nurse activates the intent to nurse. Intentional compassion energy was discovered in the meaning of the nurse participants being in their everydayness of practice. The participants described the intention to care compassionately as the grounding of their practice, striving to understand the other, to make a difference while living their nursing as an evolving process. Hermeneutic phenomenology provided the opening to discover what keeps nurses in nursing.

Contents

CHAPTER 1

INTRODUCTION

Nursing

Compassion, kindness, caring and love to [*sic*] my profession was [*sic*] what I experienced today. You see, I am one of those nurses who became a nurse because I thought nursing was a novel vocation. This week I fell in love with nursing one more time. This I owed to a patient of mine. His name is Mr. O. Mr. O. has been fighting coronary artery disease for the last 20 years. He has had multiple myocardial infarctions in the past as well. This week he came to the hospital because he has been feeling more fatigued than usual. Because of his extensive cardiac history, the nurse practitioner for whom I was working decided to admit Mr. O. I thought it was best for him to stay for a couple of days to run a few more tests and for observation. During my short encounter with him, I cared

> for him. And I made a difference in his life. I cared for his soul, body, person, dreams, ideas, and after all was done, he thanked me for being present. I went home that night feeling overwhelmed with the love I have for my profession, and how Mr. O. helped me more than I helped him. (Roccio G. Vinas, personal communication, July 1, 2008)

The above nursing situation was a journal entry from a graduate student in which she described how her nursing made a difference in her life and in her patient's, Mr. O's, life. This nursing situation inspired the question, "What keeps nurses in nursing?" Compassion, kindness, caring and love are the ingredients for this nurse. This graduate nursing student's expression of caring gives the impression of energetic love for the nursing profession. As my student, she inspired me, her clinical practice faculty, to nurture her vigor and stamina, as well as my own. Then the notions unfolded as I wondered, do all nurses fall in love with nursing each day that they nurse?

Background

The nursing shortage in the United States is a result of the aging workforce, increased professional opportunities for women, decreased enrollment in nursing programs, shortage of nursing faculty, and the aging population (American Association of

Colleges of Nursing [AACN], 2008). Several factors associated with the workplace environment result in nursing job dissatisfaction among nurses. These include violence in the workplace, understaffing, and an increase in nonnursing duties (Evans, 2005; Jackson, Clare & Mannix, 2002; O'Brien-Pallas, Duffield & Alksnis, 2004). Most of this research, however, has been investigated from a quantitative perspective and takes on a negative focus, in other words, what is wrong. Little is qualitatively known about the positive view: What keeps nurses in nursing. Research findings suggest one in five nurses will leave the workforce for reasons other than retirement (Aiken, Clarke, Sloane, Sochalski, & Silber, 2002). Annually, turnover rates for nurses have ranged from 12% in 1996, 15% in 1999, and 26% in 2000 creating increased labor recruitment costs and threatening the quality of patient care (Aiken et al., 2002; Joint Commission on Accreditation of Healthcare Organizations [JCAHO], 2004; Larrabee et al., 2003). Additionally, it is estimated that by the year 2011 the number of nurses leaving the profession will exceed the number of new nurses beginning their careers (U.S. Department of Health and Human Services, 2002).

The combined impact of these and other indicators has resulted in the implementation of retention strategies such as increased wages, educational reimbursement, flexible shifts and retention bonuses with varying degree of success (AACN, 2008; Buerhaus, 2007; Hart, 2005). Qualitatively, however, little is known about the experiences that influence the decision of nurses to stay in their current position and to what extent this experience influences nurses' retention. Studying what keeps nurses in nursing can provide insight into approaches useful for promoting retention of a quality caring and compassionate nursing workforce.

Studies convey that nurses do not have the time to provide the compassionate care they desire (Abendroth & Flannery, 2006; Cowin & Hengstberger-Sims, 2005; Sabo, 2006). Nursing is more demanding and multifaceted than it has ever been. The demand on nurses continues to increase due to patient acuity, changes in reimbursement, access to care and technology (Christmas, 2008). When a nurse was asked if she had time to provide compassionate care, she responded "I care, but I have so many things to care about, I have to ration it" (Cara S. Calloway, personal communication, March 24, 2007).

The patient's suffering may impact the ability of the nurse to be present with the nursed. When the call for the nurse is fear, pain, suffering, sadness, loss, anxiety or frustration, the nurse can perceive it as threatening. As a defense, the nurse may relate from a distance or hide behind the technical equipment, and be present with the monitor rather than with the one nursed (Johnston, 2007).

One of the top five reasons identified for the nursing shortage is a negative healthcare work environment (Buerhaus, 2007). Few would argue that nursing work is stressful. Present day nurses face many challenges in caring for the nursed.

Stress is an assumed cost of doing nursing work and may be interpreted as an individual's problem to solve (Sabo, 2006). Society, and even other nurses, judge nurses' emotional reactions to stress and patient loss harshly. Nurses' resignation towards stress and their assumption of individual responsibility may prevent identification of serious job stress that is rooted in the work place and not in the nurses' emotional state. Nurses may exit the workforce as a way to negotiate their stress as they have lost the ability to nurture and are at risk for compassion fatigue.

Time, suffering, negative healthcare work environment, and stress have been studied quantitatively in regards to the present nursing shortage. Yet, there are no qualitative studies in the literature that ask nurses about their experience and desire to care for a patient in the context of the nursing situation.

Significance

Exploring what keeps nurses in nursing will contribute to the body of nursing knowledge and practice. First hand perspective from the nurses' experiences can elicit implications for nursing practice to revise or add to the caring process. Compassionate caring can be provided for the nursed in an efficient and timely manner, to benefit the nurse and the nursed. The culture of nursing should be considered and nurtured as compassion in present day practice. Qualitative research into what keeps nurses in nursing will be emergent, interpretive and view the phenomena holistically.

The nurses' experiences can be interpreted to discover the meaning of being in the everydayness. The expression of caring work using the nurse's voice for the interpretation of the nature of her or his truth, language, thinking, dwelling, and being brings the profession to a better understanding of what it takes to continue to nurse in light of the looming nursing shortage.

Purpose

The purpose of this study was to explore what keeps nurses in nursing by examining the impact of the relational experiences between the nurse and her or his patient in the context of the nursing situation. Heideggerian hermeneutic phenomenology was the philosophy that grounded the study and the method used to interpret the nursing situation. The underlying energy of the purpose for this study inspired the research question "what keeps nurses in nursing?"

Definitions

Compassion

Fox (1979) asserts that the interdependence of human beings means that all are a part of one another and all are involved in one another. According to Fox (1979) "compassion operates at the same level as celebration. The awareness of togetherness urges us to rejoice at another's joy (celebration) and to grieve at another's sorrow" (p. 4). Celebration is considered a letting go of ego and overcoming the difficulty of entering into others' suffering in order to relieve others' suffering (Watson, 1985, 2006).

Lundberg and Boonprasabhai's (2001) ethnographic study defined compassion as giving care from the heart, valuing people, respect, trust, and loving concern. Experiencing compassion, the nurse seeks to know and understand interconnectedness to others in order to alleviate suffering and celebrate joy with the nursed (Fox, 1979; Roach, 2002). Roach (2002) defines compassion as a way of living born out of an awareness of one's relationship to all living creatures. It engenders a response of participation in the experience of another's sensitivity to the pain and brokenness of the other and a quality of presence that allows one to share with and make room for the other. (p. 50).

Compassion involves a simple, unpretentious presence with the other (Roach, 2002). A nurse's lack of presence may indicate avoidance behavior. Suffering seems to call forth a natural human tendency to distance one's self from exposure to vulnerability (Johnston, 2007). Compassion is one of the essences of care. The nurse compassionately nurtures the one nursed. The call from the nursed is heard by the nurse. The nurse response is compassionate intention in the context of the nursing situation (Boykin & Schoenhofer, 2001; Paterson & Zderad, 1988). Compassion is regarded as an active, positive emotion with volitional qualities (Johnston, 2007).

A nurse may perform actions for the one nursed with a sense of duty or moral obligation. The nurse, in this case, acts out of duty, not compassion. The value of human care and caring involves a higher sense of spirit of self (Watson, 1985). Compassion is a gift and cannot be acquired by advanced skills and techniques (Roach, 2002, p. 51). For this study, compassion was described as being present with another to alleviate suffering and celebrate joy. This description was synthesized from the work of Boykin and Schoenhofer (2001), Fox (1979), Johnston (2007), Paterson and Zderad (1988), Roach (2002), and Watson (1985).

Nurturance

Common usage defines nurturance as affectionate care and attention (Merriam-Webster, 2008). Nurturing acts are behaviors directed toward another with the intention of providing physical or psychological nourishment (Sappington, 2003). This definition illuminates how nurses care in a manner that respects the uniqueness and value of the nursed. An important dimension of a successful nurturing act requires the nurse to assess and respond to the emotions and needs of the nursed (Sappington, 2003).

Nurturance is an attribute within compassionate presence (Fox, 1979; Johnston, 2007; Roach, 2002; Watson, 1985, 2006). Quality presence transforms compassion for the nurse and nursed to promote and nurture health and well-being with each other (Newman, 1994; Roach, 2002). The nurse answers the call to nurse with the intent to know the nursed by alleviating suffering and seeking interconnectedness with the nurse (Fox, 1979; Paterson & Zderad, 1988; Roach, 2002). For this study, nurturance was described as the nourishment of affectionate care for health and well-being for both the nurse and the nursed. This definition was synthesized from the work of Boykin and Schoenhofer (2001), Fox (1979), Johnston (2007), Newman (1994), Roach (2002), Sappington (2003), and Watson (1985, 2006).

Energy

Once the nurse answers the call of the nursed compassionately and with the intention of alleviating suffering, an interaction of energy occurs (Boykin & Schoenhofer, 2001; Fox, 1979; Newman, 1994; Paterson & Zderad, 1988; Roach, 2002). In the Science of Unitary Human Beings, Rogers' describes energy fields as continuously open, infinite, dynamic and integral. The energies of person and environment flow continuously through each other in unbroken waves (Newman, 1994; Rogers, 1970). The mutual patterning manifestations reflect the unpredictable field changes flowing in lower and higher frequencies (Todaro-Franceschi, 1999). The process of field changes that continually fluctuate are essential to wholeness and rhythmical patterning (Malinski, 2006).

Human energy fields are inseparable and infinitely transcend space and time, forever actualizing potentials (Rogers,

1970; Todaro-Franceschi, 1999). Creative and innovative potentials promote well being of the nurse and nursed by resonating at a centering frequency (Newman, 1994; Rogers, 1970; Todaro-Franceschi, 1999). The human experience is a process of expanding consciousness to recognize the power within a person that moves her or him to a higher level of consciousness (Newman, 1994).

Information about feeling and meaning of the nursed emerges from the underlying patterns of energy (Newman, 2008). Pattern recognition happens in the context of a nursing situation, which is centered on exploring that which is most meaningful (Boykin & Schoenhofer, 2001; Pharris, 2006). Energy patterning depicts the relational interaction within the nursing situation.

Newman (1994, 2008) views energy as a dynamic process resulting in transformative purposeful change. Each person's energy field is expressed in unique patterns. The human and environmental energy fields are dynamic and exist in an integral and infinite mutual process (Newman 1994, 2008; Rogers, 1970).

The nurse's energy pattern becomes vibrational and resonates at a centering frequency (Todaro-Franceschi, 1999). The patient's energy pattern initially resonates at lower frequency then moves towards the higher energy frequency of the nurse. The nurse and the nursed connect at one resonant pulsating centered frequency. The nurse and the nursed then are transformed to a higher level of consciousness (Newman, 2008, p. 34). The relationship between the nurse and nursed continues until the nursed finds his or her own rhythmic vibration from which both the nurse and nursed experience the other (Newman, 1994, 2008; Rogers, 1970). For this study, energy was described as mutual patterning manifestation unpredictable field changes that resonate from lower to higher frequencies resulting in a higher level of consciousness. This definition was synthesized from the work of Newman (1994, 2008), Rogers (1970), and Todaro-Franceschi (1999).

Intentionality

The intention of nurses is to nurture a person (Boykin & Schoenhofer, 2001). Henderson (1961) defines nursing as assisting the individual, sick or well, in the performance of those activities contributing to health or its recovery (or a peaceful death) that he would perform unaided if he had the necessary strength, will, or knowledge. And to do this in such a way as to help the individual gain independence as rapidly as possible (p. 42).

Common usage defines intentionality as the property of being about or directed toward a subject, as inherent in conscious states, beliefs, or creations of the mind (American Heritage Dictionary of the English Language, 2006). Intentionality and authentic presence allow the nurse to hear the call (Boykin & Schoenhofer, 2001; Paterson & Zderad, 1988). The nurse enters into the nursing situation with the intentional commitment of knowing the patient as a caring person. Intentionality in the nursing situation has the potential to promote energy flow to both nurse and nursed (Boykin & Schoenhofer, 2001; Paterson & Zderad, 1988; Rogers, 1970).

Using intention, the nursing response is a caring expression of nurturing to sustain, enhance and energize the nurse and nursed in the nursing situation (Boykin & Schoenhofer, 2001; Newman, 2008). The nursing response is uniquely created and unpredictable in the moment (Todaro-Franceschi, 1999).

In the caring-between the nurse and nursed, energy processing is initiated and personhood is enhanced (Boykin & Schoenhofer, 2001; Newman, 2008; Paterson & Zderad, 1988). As the nurse intentionally comes to know self as caring, she or he lets go of ego to experience the interconnectedness that enables the nurse to know self and other as living and caring (Boykin & Schoenhofer, 2001; Watson, 1985, 2006).

Intentionality promotes a healing caring consciousness as energy within the human environment field of a caring moment (Watson, 2006). Watson (2006) states that "cultivation of sensitivity to one's self and to others becomes a cultivation of one's own spiritual practices and transpersonal self, going beyond ego self, opening to others with sensitivity and compassion" (p. 298). In a caring consciousness, nurse and nursed experience a subtle energy environment whereby compassionate love and caring come together intentionally to form a deep transpersonal caring occasion (Watson, 1985).

Nursing has an ethical-theoretical-philosophical orientation known as the caritas processes (Watson, 2006). The nurse is viewed as a co-participant in the human care process with high value placed on the relationship between the nurse and the nursed (Watson, 1985, p. 35). When the nurse answers the call of the nursed with the intent to alleviate suffering; the nursed reveals her or his hopes, dreams and aspirations. The nurse's and nursed's individual expressions of affirmation, support and celebration are exchanged as energy via compassionate presence (Locsin, 2006, p. 386). Compassion becomes the energy of caring (Johns, 2005).

In the nursing situation, the nurse answers the call with patterned nurturance which yields energy to be compassionately present. The dynamic unfolding of the energy exchange is experienced as patterned nurturance through listening, knowing and being with the nursed in authentic compassionate presence (Swanson, 1991; Watson, 2006). In the context of the nursing situation, there is a vibrational centering which is meaningful and nourishes nurturance. This energy patterning is depicted as patterned nurturance (Todaro-Franceschi, 1999).

In intentional caring consciousness, the nurse intentionally knows the nursed as whole. The patient has the choice of letting the nurse know her or him as person (Boykin & Schoenhofer, 2001; Locsin, 1998). For this study, intentionality was described as purposefully assisting the nursed towards promoting a healing and healthy consciousness. This definition was synthesized from Boykin & Schoenhofer (2001), Paterson & Zderad (1988), and Watson (2006).

Compassion Energy

Nurses initiate the experience of compassion energy when they answer the call from a patient. The three attributes of compassion energy are compassionate presence, patterned nurturance, and intentionally knowing the nursed and self as whole (Dunn, 2007).

When the nurse answers the call of the nursed with the intent to alleviate suffering or celebrate joy, the nursed reveals her or his hopes, dreams, and aspirations. The nurse and the nursed's individual expressions of affirmation, support, and celebration are exchanged as energy via compassionate presence. Compassion becomes the energy of caring (Dunn, 2007).

In the nursing situation, the nurse answers the call with patterned nurturance that yields energy to be compassionately present. The dynamic unfolding of the energy exchange is experienced as patterned nurturance through listening, knowing, and being with the nursed in authentic presence. In the context of the nursing situation, there is a vibrational centering that is meaningful and nourishes nurturance. This energy patterning is depicted as patterned nurturance (Dunn, 2007; Todaro-Franceschi, 1999).

In intentional caring consciousness, the nurse intentionally knows the nursed as whole. Compassion energy is the intersubjective gift of compassion that gives nurses the opportunity to be with the nursed. Alleviating suffering or celebrating joy, the nurse and the nursed express a warm approval while sharing joyful satisfaction in the nursing situation by enhancing compassionate presence, patterned nurturance, and intentionally knowing the nursed and self as whole (Dunn, 2007).

Nurses who self-generate vigor as compassion energy find meaning in caring for others. When nurses self-generate vigor, they regenerate the capacity to foster interconnectedness with the nursed. Compassion energy is defined as the regeneration of nurses' capacity to foster interconnectedness when the nurse activates the intent to nurse (Dunn, 2007).

Theoretical Perspective

The theoretical framework of Boykin and Schoenhofer's Nursing as Caring Theory (NAC; 2001) was used to explore what keeps nurses in nursing. The unified attribute for this research was caring. Boykin and Schoenhofer posit the unique focus of nursing as nurturing persons living caring and growing in caring. A person is enhanced by being part of a nurturing relationship with a caring person. As the nurse intentionally comes to know self as caring, she or he lets go of ego to experience the interconnectedness that enables the nurse to know self and other as living caring. The nurse answers the call to nurse with the intent to know the one nursed by alleviating suffering and seeking interconnectedness with the one nursed (Roach, 2002). Once the nurse answers the call of the nursed compassionately, and with the intention of alleviating suffering, an interaction of energy occurs (Newman, 1994; Rogers, 1970). Nurses enhance personhood by participating in nurturing relationships with caring others in the moment (Boykin & Schoenhofer, 2001).

The nursing situation is the place in which to dwell to discover knowledge and enhance personhood. The theory of Nursing as Caring offers a view that inspires a broad, encompassing understanding of any and all situations of nursing practice. Boykin and Schoenhofer (2006) state that certain fundamental beliefs of what it means to be human reflect values that provide a basis for understanding and explicating the meaning of nursing. Nursing as Caring assumptions and key themes are as follows: persons are caring by virtue of their humanness; persons are whole and complete in the moment; persons live caring from moment to moment; personhood is enhanced through participation in nurturing relationships with caring others; and nursing is both a discipline and a profession (Boykin & Schoenhofer, 2006). Nurses as Caring Theory assumptions provide an organizing value system and perspective to explore meaning and understanding of nurses' work.

Compassion is one of the essences of care. The nurse compassionately nurtures the nursed. The call from the nursed is heard by the nurse. The nurse response is compassionate intention in the context of the nursing situation (Boykin & Schoenhofer, 2001). Roach (2002) states that "caring is the unique manifestation of a person being-in-the-world" (p. 30). The human expression of caring can be revealed through compassion or love, sorrow or joy, sadness or despair in the caring-between the nurse and the nursed.

In the caring-between the nurse and nursed, an energy exchange is initiated and personhood is enhanced (Boykin & Schoenhofer, 2001; Newman, 2008; Paterson & Zderad, 1988; Rogers, 1970). Thus, the nurse is viewed as a co-participant in the human care process with high value placed on the relationship between the nurse and the nursed (Watson, 1985, p. 35).

Researcher's Perspective

> I was overdue for lunch and hungry when LC arrived, pale, diaphoretic, holding his chest with one hand and grabbing my arm with his other. The nursing call was loud and clear, 'call my wife and don't let me die'. Lunch and hunger were no more. Compassion became the feast. (Dunn, 2007)

In the above nursing situation, I discovered revitalization in the call of the one nursed that enhanced my personhood (Boykin &

Schoenhofer, 2001). My compassion for LC led me to discover a source of energy. Through this process, it is possible for other nurses to generate or regenerate compassion within her or his capacity to foster interconnectedness.

For this researcher, nursing has been a source of economic survival and a source of personal growth and love. Nurses confronted with high intellectual, emotional, and physical job demands and have low intellectual, emotional, and physical job resources are at risk for physical complaints, compassion fatigue, and burnout (van den Tooren & de Jonge, 2008, p. 82). The nursing situation is an interactive qualitative place to dwell and study the dynamic and evolving energetic process of compassion. The nursing situation is a natural setting for nursing research (Boykin & Schoenhofer, 2001). The aim is to understand perspectives, perceptions, meaning, and uniqueness of the subjective lives of the nurse and nursed and what is occurring between them in the encounter. The researcher attends to the temporal, social and historical contexts of the nursing situation. For the nurse, in the context of the nursing situation, the meaning and purpose were explored through an interpretive phenomenological exploration of what is it that keeps the nurse nursing at the bedside, curbside, under trees, or wherever nursing takes place.

Chapter Summary

In Chapter 1, I introduced the question—do all nurses fall in love with nursing again and again? In the background, there was a description of the nursing shortage qualitative research gap in the literature. The significance section explained the importance of conducting this study qualitatively. The purpose of this study included a discussion of the research questions. The theoretical perspective was briefly introduced and grounds the study that is further developed in Chapter 3. The researcher's perspective, both as a practicing nurse and nurse researcher, was explained.

CHAPTER 2

REVIEW OF THE LITERATURE

This chapter provides a review of the literature regarding what keeps nurses in nursing. The first section is a description of care and caring, followed by a discussion of caring work from the perspective of professional satisfaction, which describes the culture of nursing. A review of burnout and compassion fatigue is presented. Lastly, compassion in nursing concludes this chapter.

Care and Caring

Kramer's (1974) quasi-experimental study exposed "why nurses leave nursing" in her discovery of the concept described as "reality shock." Reality shock occurs when new graduates encounter the real life differences between their perceptions of what nursing should be and the actual reality of the workplace. Kramer suggested that reality shock can manifest as hopelessness and dissatisfaction, which are preludes to conflict in the workplace.

Unfortunately, professional bureaucratic conflicts in nursing continue into the 21st century. Nurses' disillusionment with hospital workforce management is threatening the provision of care. Caring research has evolved during the past 20 years; however, the concept of caring may have more than one possible meaning or interpretation (Baer, 1992; Kramer, 1974; Ray & Turkel, 2002).

Finfgeld-Connett's (2006) meta-synthesis of caring from 49 qualitative studies and six concept analyses of caring provides an understanding of what is involved for caring to take place within the nursing situation. Caring is an interpersonal process that is characterized by expert nursing practice, interpersonal sensitivity, and intimate relationships. Antecedents to the caring process include a need for and openness to caring from the patient. The nurse's precondition of the caring process consists of professional maturity and moral underpinnings. Also, a working environment conducive to caring is necessary to enhance mental well-being among patients and nurses, and improvements in patients' physical well-being (p. 198). In an evolutionary concept analysis, Brilowski and Wendler (2004) identified five core attributes of caring to include relationship, action, attitude, acceptance, and variability. Other related concepts that they identified included nurturing, compassion, concern and ministering. These related concepts were embedded in the discussion of caring in this study.

Smith (1999) analyzed caring concepts from the literature and synthesized caring concepts within the theoretical perspective of Rogers' Science of Unitary Human Beings (SUHB) using a caring concept clarification process. Smith identified the synthesis of five constitutive meanings in the Science of Unitary Human Beings: manifesting intention, attuning to dynamic flow, appreciating pattern, experiencing the infinite, and inviting creative emergence.

Nursing has put forth efforts toward recognizing the complexity and significance of the concepts of care and caring, yet caring as a concept remains elusive. Many scholars have attempted to define caring, components of care, and the processes of caring. But, instead of enlightening the reader, examination of the literature only increases confusion (Brilowski & Wendler, 2004; Finfgeld-Connett, 2006; Hudacek, 2008; Morse, Solberg, Neander, Bottoroff, & Johnson, 1990; Sherwood, 1997a; Smith, 1999).

Caring Work

The changes in healthcare delivery around the globe have intensified nurses' responsibilities and workloads. Nurses must find ways to preserve their caring practice. Caring theory informs nurses to nurture professional values. Upholding caring values in nurses' practice helps the nurse to transcend from a state where nursing is perceived as "just a job" to one of professional satisfaction. With such a mind set, the nurse will learn that to provide compassion to ease patients' and families' suffering, and to promote health, will contribute to expansion of the nurse's own actualization. Ideally, nurses attempt to make an intentional conscious effort to care for self, and the patient and family, compassionately. From the outset of modern nursing, nurses learned Nightingale's concept of environment as healing space that can expand the patient's awareness and consciousness promoting wholeness and healing to the mind-body-spirit (Nightingale, 1859/1992).

Caring work is included in the relationship between nurses, patients and their families, encompassing the mental, emotional and physical effects involved in looking after, responding to and supporting others. This relationship requires the nurse to be fully present with and for the patient and family. Within the relationship, a space is created for the patient and family to give voice and meaning to life experiences. However, when the nurse's ability to create meaning does not occur due to lack of resources, increased workload or tension between the competing philosophical beliefs of the nursing discipline, the individual nurse and the healthcare system, nurses experience stress.

Nurses may become overwhelmed with the pain and suffering and their overall health and well-being may become compromised. Repeated exposure to pain and suffering, failed attempts to alleviate that suffering, moral and ethical distress, and even death may arise within the paradigmatic conflict of the modern healthcare system. If the stress continues unabated, nurses may become vulnerable to adverse psychological effects such as those reflected in compassion fatigue, burnout and/or vicarious traumatization (Sabo, 2008). Numerous theories have been put forward to explain the results of caring work, yet little agreement exists about the nature of adverse consequences of caring work. Some researchers argue that stressed nurses are experiencing burnout (Byrne & McMurray, 1997; Kelly, Ross, Gray, & Smith, 2000; Leiter & Laschinger, 2006; Papadatou, Anagnostopoulos & Monos, 1994). Others claim that nurses may be experiencing compassion fatigue (Clark & Giorgio, 1998; Collins & Long, 2003; Keidel, 2002; Meadors & Lamson, 2008). Still others suggest vicarious traumatization (Sinclair & Hamill, 2007).

Trauma research suggests that interpersonal relationships, particularly ones in which compassion and emotional energy are fundamental attributes, as in the nurse-patient-family relationship, may play a role in the development of compassion fatigue (Figley, 2002) or vicarious traumatization (McCann & Pearlman, 1990; Pearlman, 1998). In providing assistance to patients experiencing pain, suffering or trauma, nurses may experience adverse effects similar to those of their patients (Valent, 2002). Conversely, research on work life and the work environment has demonstrated that the relationship may not play a central role in the onset of burnout (Lee & Ashforth, 1996).

Job Stress

Implicit in patient care is the nurse's interpersonal and empathic connection with patients and their families. Nurses' continual negotiation among professional standards, personal ego, integrity and patient needs within the nurse-patient-family relationship, and the larger healthcare system, leave the nurse vulnerable to stress, compassion fatigue, and burnout. Nurses' effective use of self-care techniques contribute to improved patient care and increased job satisfaction (Aiken et al., 2002; Haalbesleben, Wakefield, Wakefield, & Cooper, 2008; Luquette, 2007).

Research links stress to physiological conditions like cardiovascular distress, immunosuppression and gastrointestinal problems. Stress adversely impacts attention, concentration, critical thinking, and other cognitive functions. Family and social relations suffer. Staff stress levels contribute to reduced patient satisfaction, increased employee health costs, increased spending for nurse recruiting and unnecessary turnover of nurse employees (Buerhaus, Donelan, Ulrich, Norman & Dittus, 2006; Halldorsdottir, 2007; Latham, Hogan, & Ringl, 2008; Raup, 2008).

In a longitudinal study over three years, Gelsema et al. (2006) examined the causes and consequences of job stress in 381 hospital nurses. Gelsema et al. discovered that a change in work conditions is predictive of stress outcomes, especially of job satisfaction and emotional exhaustion.

The literature is limited on work stress that addresses the relationship between stressors of nursing work and the effect on the well-being of nurses.

Rose and Glass (2006), using a qualitative critical feminist research inquiry of five female community mental health nurses in Australia, investigated the relationship between emotional well-being and effective functioning as community mental health nurses. The participants revealed a strong relationship between satisfying professional practice and positive emotional well-being and, equally, dissatisfying professional satisfaction and negative emotional well-being.

A combination of stress management and self-care interventions appear to be more effective than any single intervention to support nurses' well-being. Providing multiple self-care techniques minimizes the consequences of stress, promotes better patient care, and increases job satisfaction (Gelsema et al., 2006; Luquette, 2007; Rose & Glass, 2006).

In interviews with 168 nurses, Simms, Erbin-Roesemann, Darga, and Coeling (1990) explored work excitement in nursing to describe nurses who do well and enjoy their work. Work excitement was defined by Simms et al. (1990) as, "personal enthusiasm and commitment for work, evidenced by creativity, receptivity to learning and ability to see opportunity in everyday situations" (p. 178). Jensen, Beck-Petterson, and Segesten (1993) described green-thumb phenomena in nurses, found in nurses who have an inner power that helps others grow and flourish in spite of a difficult health situation. These researchers conducted semi-structured interviews with 16 nurses. Three main concepts were identified as characteristic of the green-thumb phenomena: competence, compassion, and courage.

The profession of nursing is struggling to identify the professional practice environment best suited to support the nurse and ensure success in managing more complex and acute patient care. The nature of most healthcare organizations has evolved into a bureaucratic one, in which decisions are made at a level higher than the point of service. This results in a work environment that is not conducive to fostering the autonomy that the professional nurse requires to retain professional integrity and obtain positive patient outcomes. Many healthcare institutions have made efforts to restructure the practice environment and increase the autonomy and decision making authority of the nurse. Studies have demonstrated that an improved practice environment with higher levels of autonomy result in increased nurse job satisfaction (American Nurses Association [ANA], 2001; Lee & Cummings, 2008).

Job satisfaction has been defined as a feeling, experience and expectation of what a job should be, based on personal and work related factors. Lee and Cummings (2008) suggest that job satisfaction could be thought of as the attainment of needs according to Maslow’s hierarchy. Each study has a different interpretation or conceptualization of job satisfaction. A comparison between executive, frontline management level nurses and staff nurses required further research to examine factors that affect satisfaction at various levels of organization and managerial levels. Factors that satisfy managers at one level may not satisfy nurses at other levels (Lee & Cummings, 2008).

Today's nursing shortages are unlike any that have gone before and this scarcity is expected to grow through the first quarter of the 21st century. The current crisis has been caused by fundamental paradigm shifts in society and in the healthcare industry. These shifts include a decrease in the relative attractiveness of healthcare delivery, increased competition from employers in other sectors of the economy, as well as demographic and population changes (ANA, 2001; Buerhaus, 2008; Gelinas & Bohlen, 2002).

Fifty-six percent of nurses surveyed by the American Nurses Association stated that their available work time for direct patient care has decreased over a 2-year period. Consequently, 75% of nurses sampled think that the quality of nursing care at the facility in which they work has been compromised. Nearly 27% of nurses say they feel exhausted and discouraged by nursing care (ANA, 2001).

Aiken, Clarke, Sloane, and Sochalski's (2001) staff dissatisfaction study of 43,000 nurses in 711 hospitals in five countries revealed that low levels of nurse morale are a global problem (p. 43). In the U.S., more than 40% of nurses working in hospitals reported job dissatisfaction, with more than 43% demonstrating high levels of burnout. Twenty-three percent of nurses in the U.S. said they planned to leave their current job in the next year. This figure was higher (33%) for nurses under the age of 30, as they planned to leave their current job in the next year (Aiken et al., 2001, p. 46).

Many rewards and difficulties exist for nurses who provide care to a suffering patient. Overtime, work, employee, job, and task semantics have infiltrated the nursing literature, making invisible nurses concern for the patient, the caring and the nurturance known as the human relation element in the work environment. A smaller body of literature exists regarding nurses who do well in their work. Topics and themes of nurses who are happy in their work include work excitement (Simms et al., 1990); competence, compassion, and courage (Jensen et al., 1993); and caring spirituality (Zerwekh, 1993).

Unit Culture

Research has shown a link between healthy work cultures and healthy employees. Ideally, nurses are compassionate, caring individuals who need to know about the culture of their work environment. The literature on work unit culture reveals that, depending on the workgroup culture, employees will respond emotionally to the dynamics of a working nursing unit as they occur. Each nursing unit has its own unique culture that influences the dynamics of the unit. The culture of a work environment matters because employees and employers make decisions based on the cultural forces operating in that environment which, if not anticipated, may have undesirable consequences (Hawkins & Kratsch, 2004; Mulcahy & Betts, 2005; Schein, 1999; Sirgo & Coeling, 2005).

Mulcahy and Betts (2005) investigated unit culture in relation to the retention of neonatal nurses. They utilized cultural mapping techniques that revealed beliefs different for each professional group. Strong subcultures existed in the unit among new nurse groups, less experienced nurse groups and more experienced nurse groups. The researchers determined that, if the culture is negative and non-supportive, it will negatively impact the health of the nurse employee.

There are gaps in the literature regarding the combination of nursing unit culture, work stress, and their relationship to the sense of well-being of nurses. Gifford, Zammuto, and Goodman (2002) investigated the relationship between unit organizational culture and job-related variables for nurse retention in the labor and delivery units of seven hospitals. The findings suggested that improving quality of work life is a practical and long term approach to improving nurse retention. This body of research generally considers the relationship between job-related factors and nurse retention (Beaudoin & Edgar, 2003; Gardiner, Sexton,

Durbridge & Garrard, 2005; Gifford et al., 2002). The majority of the available literature exists within the psychology and occupational health literature, rather than the nursing literature.

The study of unit culture and work stress in nursing is relatively new; therefore insight gained from this present study will expand the body of existing nursing research. Most studies of nurses and stress have relied on the use of instruments that measure burnout in human service personnel. Research instruments from the business and psychosocial disciplines measure culture and compassion fatigue and an attempt to use these instruments in nursing may add to the confusion (Figley, 2002; Gelsema et al., 2006).

Burnout and Compassion Fatigue

Freudenberger (1974) developed the expression burnout in cognitive, physical and behavioral terms. McCarthy (1985), in an examination of burnout in psychiatric nurses, defined burnout as "a syndrome characterized by progressive physical and emotional exhaustion involving the development of negative job attitudes and perceptions and a loss of empathetic concern for patients. Burnout is caused by chronic emotional stress from the prolonged involvement with people" (p. 305). Maslach (1982) defined burnout as a psychological response to work-related stress that consists of: emotional exhaustion (a depletion of work-related emotional resources); depersonalization (pulling away from those associated with the job); and, reduced perceptions of personal accomplishments (a belief that one is not as good at the job as he or she once was). Burnout has become an important concern for healthcare organizations because of its negative consequences in terms of turnover, job satisfaction and performance (Aiken et al., 2002; Haalbesleben & Buckley, 2004). Burnout literature describes the underlying causes without attention to consequences of burnout. It has become common to assume that burnout has significant negative consequences (Haalbesleben et al., 2008).

Joinson (1992) was the first to use the term compassion fatigue while studying burnout in nurses working in emergency departments. Joinson (1992) described compassion fatigue as being vertically ill. Vertically ill was defined as functioning but not attending to the nurse's own emotional needs. The nurse risked the loss of the ability to nurture. Nurses at risk for compassion fatigue are described as empathetic, caring individuals who may absorb the traumatic stress of those they help. Often the duration of the experience is a factor as well as exposure to death, dying or destruction (Figley, 1995;

Joinson, 1992

Figley (1995) described compassion fatigue as a natural consequence of behaviors and emotions resulting from knowing about a traumatizing event experienced by a significant other. Compassion fatigue is the stress resulting from helping or wanting to help a traumatized or suffering person. The contrary construct is the nurse who is unable to be present with the traumatized or suffering person and, as a result, may exhibit avoidance behavior.

According to Figley (2002), educators in the caring professions have a special obligation to students to prepare them for the hazards of stress, burnout and compassion fatigue. Figley (2002) suggested the addition of compassion fatigue to nursing curricula because of its acute onset. Compassion fatigue is a known stressor in nursing which can lead to burnout and may coexist with burnout. Compassion fatigue has emerged as a natural consequence of caring for those who are in pain, suffering or traumatized (Figley, 1995). Authors express interest in how nursing work and caring might impact the health of nurses and their presence with another (Abrenroth & Flannery, 2006; Sabo, 2006). Nurses are at risk for denying physical, social, emotional and spiritual needs for self. The nurse can be traumatized or suffer through her or his own efforts to empathize and be compassionate. This can lead to poor self-care and extreme self-sacrifice in the process of caring for the nursed. The nurse is then at risk for suffering from compassion fatigue (Dunn, 2005).

Sabo (2008) described compassion fatigue as different from burnout. Compassion fatigue is acute, usually limited to a duration of three weeks. Burnout is chronic and can last from months to years. Although compassion fatigue is a "new" hazard to nurses' health, there are no current psychometric instruments to accurately measure the phenomenon in nurses. Since Joinson (1992) coined the term compassion fatigue and Figley (2002) described the phenomenon, it has remained obscure in the healthcare literature. Recently, compassion fatigue has been exposed as a symptom of stress in caregivers but the literature review yielded relatively few studies. Some studies (Adams, Figley & Boscarmo, 2008; Clark & Giorgio 1998; Collins & Long, 2003; Sabo, 2006; Schwarz, 2005) addressed the detrimental effects of the phenomenon on the health of caregivers such as policemen, trauma rescue workers, and social workers. Although there have been observations of compassion fatigue in nurses, no studies were found that focus on the relationship between compassion fatigue and the well-being of nurses. The scarcity of nurse-related research in this area supports the need for research evidence to explain anecdotal observations. Presently compassion fatigue is known as a stress response that is sudden and acute and is defined as a physical, emotional and spiritual fatigue or exhaustion that takes over a person, causing a decline in her or his ability to experience joy or care for others (McMullen, 2007).

Compassion in Nursing

Compassion plays an essential role in the perceptions of consumers of healthcare and their experience of the quality of nursing care. Despite this perception of compassion in nursing, the review of literature for compassion revealed there is little known in the professional literature that addresses the essences of compassion as experienced by nurses.

Compassion, empathy and loving concern transform lives. Nurses desire to provide compassionate care. In the early 1900s, Lavinia L. Dock, Lillian D. Wald, and Annie W. Goodrich considered compassion not only as the essence of nursing, but also an inherent quality a nurse should have (Hamilton, 1994). Common public perception expects nurses to have more compassionate impulses than other people, or act on them more often. In such sentiments, the nurse is expected to be constantly compassionate and caring as part of the job. The institutionalization of compassion can make it routine and devoid of feeling. Even if the impulse of compassion attracts people to nursing, it is not always translated into action. In the past, improving quality care meant focusing on racial and geographic disparities, patient safety and adherence to clinical guidelines, but not compassion. Most interventions to improve compassion primarily target students. What is missing is a method to continually reinforce the positive aspects of compassion among practicing registered nurses (Salvage, 2006; Sanghavi, 2006).

Lundberg & Boonprasabhai (2001) ethnographic study of 20 Thai female nursing students in their last year described the meaning and practical expression of good nursing care. The six categories that emerged were: compassion, competency, communication, comfort, creation and courage. Compassion was described as giving care from the heart, valuing people, respect, trust, and loving concern.

In the past two decades, scholars have been redefining nursing in the nurse-patient-family relationship, emphasizing intimacy as its vehicle for effective delivery of care. The previous biomedical structures, disease labeling and technological tasks have fostered an environment which has made it possible to practice detachment under the banner of professionalism (Sanghavi, 2006).

Sanghavi (2006) reviewed questionnaires and transcripts of Schwartz rounds from multidiscipline caregivers at 54 hospitals in 21 states. The review yielded three strong common themes, communication, common ground and respect for individuality. The most frequently cited suggestion to improve compassionate care focused on body language and content of communication. Participants expressed that caregivers could make a conscious choice to care deeply for patients.

Peters (2006) qualitative phenomenological study of eleven nurse faculty members offered insights into the lifeworld of faculty members' experience of compassion. The themes that emerged were that compassion begins with forming connections with others that enable faculty to 'walk a mile in their shoes' living their suffering as if it were their own. The faculty members described an initiation of action to alleviate suffering with a willingness to go beyond what is expected, giving the gift of self, time, or actions for the person in need. In giving this gift, often, faculty received a gift in return.

Schantz (2007) concept analysis clarified the meaning of compassion and its relevance in the context of everyday nursing practice. Nurses make a conscious decision to choose compassion in nursing decisions and actions and as an inspiration to achieve excellence in everyday nursing practice. Yet, the concept of compassion is hardly found in connection with contemporary nursing literature. Caring, sympathy and empathy are found generously within nursing literature. The literature implies that these words are being used interchangeably with compassion. Compassion empowers nurses. Many nurses will say it is compassion for others that inspired them to become a nurse.

The literature suggest nursing curriculum that addresses educating nurses to be with others in a compassionate way. Younger (1990) suggest that meaning and struggles discovered through literary works can expand nursing students' knowledge concerning the experience of others living with adversity. Other scholars describe ways for nurses to care for self to regenerate the need to facilitate effective nurse-patient-family relationships characterized by compassionate caring. What is needed is a method to continuously reinforce compassion for nursing students and all professional nurses (Dunn, 2008; Manteso, 2005; Salvage, 2006; Sanghavi, 2006).

Chapter Summary

There are gaps in the literature regarding the combination of unit culture, work stress, compassion fatigue and their relationship to the sense of well-being of nurses. Some studies demonstrate the relationship strain among organizational cultures, subcultures and employee well-being. However, there is a notable absence of recent studies in the nursing literature linking unit culture, work stress and compassion fatigue. Compassion in nursing literature represents the barriers and challenges nurses confront to actually be able to provide desired compassionate care. The literature review supports the need for further nursing research into the question: what keeps nurses in nursing.

CHAPTER 3

METHODOLOGY

This chapter presents a description of the method for this qualitative study. Qualitative research methods guide the exploration of everyday experiences. Specifically, Heideggerian hermeneutic phenomenology was used to explore and interpret what keeps nurses in nursing. There is a discussion of the ethical considerations, the participants, and approach to data collection, analysis, interpretation and methodological rigor.

Method

Edmund Husserl (1859-1939) is considered the founder of phenomenology. For Husserl, the aim of phenomenology is a description of how the world is constituted and experienced through consciousness (Husserl, 1967). The goal of phenomenology is a descriptive, detached analysis of consciousness in which objects are constituted (Embree, 2006).

Husserl (1967) declared that experience is the source of all knowledge and to describe ones experience would only be possible by bracketing the assumptions of the investigator, to remove them from contaminating data. Husserl introduced the notion of the lived experience, presupposed the mind-body duality of Cartesian philosophy and sought to use bracketing as a way of removing presuppositions (Koch 1995).

Martin Heidegger (1889-1976) was a student of Husserl who rejected the notion that we are observing subjects separated from the worlds of objects about which we seek to gain knowledge; rather, he argued that we are beings inseparable from an already existing world (Draucker, 1999). For Heidegger, the essence of phenomenology is ontological and answers the questions: What is it like to be? What is being? What is being in the world? *Daisin* is the term Heidegger assigned to human beings and the term connotes being-in–the-world. Being there, for *Daisin*, defines the nature of human beings' place in context and in culture. Heidegger sought to understand life in the historical context of its developing world view (Heidegger, 1962). This is different from Husserlian phenomenology, yet resembles it to the extent of involving a sort of suspension of the everyday understanding of what it means to experience being-in-the-world (Dreyfus, 1994). *Daesin* asks the ontological question and seeks to understand the meaning of being. But, in order to arrive at the ontological meaning of being, one must first come to understand her or his own being and how she or he lives in the world (Heidegger, 1962).

According to Heidegger (1962) the lives of human beings are situated within activities and relationships that are meaningful. Situated-in–the-world means that we understand who we are through our lived experience. This understanding of who we are is seen and understood in everyday experiences. Heidegger believes there is commonality in this understanding with all other human beings. Some of these understandings may be culturally specific, or specific to the community or the individual. Being situated also means being situated at a specific point in history. Heidegger's (1962) calls our basic activity being-in-the-world as we are constantly adapting to our situation.

Heidegger takes an ontological interpretative turn from Husserl's epistemological descriptive understanding (Welch, 1999, p. 236). As the investigator of this study, I believe that bracketing is a misleading view of the processes occurring in interpretive research and argue that it separates the event from one's understanding of it (Welch, 1999). Heigdegger's emphasis is on understanding more than describing. Experiences can be understood in terms of one's background and the social context of the experiences (Draucker, 1999). The philosophical view of Heidegger posits that humans are self-interpreting, that is, they are always in the process of creating meanings from situations in which they are involved. Hermeneutics is an approach to inquiry that focuses on examining common, everyday experiences for shared meanings and practical wisdom. Phenomenology becomes hermeneutical when its method is taken to be interpretive, rather than purely descriptive as in Husserl's transcendental phenomenology (Polkinghorne, 1983). This orientation is evident in the work of Heidegger who argues that all description is always already interpretation and every form of human awareness is interpretive. In Heidegger's later work he increasingly introduces poetry and art as expressive works for interpreting the nature of truth, language, thinking, dwelling, and being (Heidegger, 1977).

Friederich Schleiermacher (1768-1834) attempted to systematize hermeneutics into one comprehensive hermeneutical philosophy in the late 18th and early 19th centuries (Polkinghorne, 1983, p. 31). Dilthey (1813-1911) was the first to appropriate hermeneutics for human science. Dilthey (1944/1976) changed the meaning of hermeneutics as he took the operations that produced understanding of texts to operations that produced knowledge of the human realm (Polkinghorne, 1983). There is a relation of parts to the whole, in which the parts receive meaning from the whole and the whole receives sense from the parts so that the movement from whole to parts to whole becomes the hermeneutic circle (Dithey, 1976; Packer, 1989; Polkinghorne, 1983). The core principle of hermeneutics is that understanding is a process that is achieved by comparison. The researcher compared a part of the text with the whole. The meaning of the text is compared with the historical or situatedness of the participant. The text is also compared with the researcher's own background. Understanding, therefore, was of a circular nature (Packer, 1989).

Method for Nursing

Heideggerian hermeneutic phenomenology guided this study as the investigator explored and interpreted the lived experience of what keeps nurses in nursing. The findings illuminated and made visible the meanings embedded in the text.

The contextualization of a situation differs among people based upon the meaning and understanding of the situation. One means for fully discovering meaning is hermeneutic phenomenology. Hermeneutic phenomenology, or hermeneutics, is a method to study how nurses interpret their lives and make meaning of what they experience (Cohen, Kahn & Steeves, 2000, p.5). Although many approaches to qualitative research exist, Heideggerian hermeneutic phenomenology provided one of the most powerful approaches to understanding the experiences of what keeps nurses in nursing.

Benner's (1984) germinal work used the ontological interpretive approach to manage the rich description of actual nursing practice (p.39). Dreyfus (1994) declared that phenomenology enables nurses to understand human beings in their physical and cultural diversity while engaging in caring practices (Benner, 1984). Benner and Wrubel (1989) state that to understand a given culture one must seek common, everyday, shared meaning. Diekelmann and Allen (1989) developed a seven stage hermeneutical, interpretive approach for analysis of transcribed interviews, which will be discussed later in this chapter. Nurse researchers have contributed to the discussion of constitutive relationships between theory and practice through a Heideggerian hermeneutic phenomenology.

The three essential tenets of Heideggerian hermeneutic phenomenology are: human beings are self-interpreting, understanding of everyday practices and understand experiences of that practice (Dreyfus, 1994). As the investigator for this research I had a tri-focal lens through which I interpreted the texts authentically. The first focus is as an experienced practicing nurse. I used the language of nursing to explore themes of the lived experience of the practicing nurse participants. The second focus is as an educator of practicing nurses to understand everyday practices, and the third focus is as a nurse scholar to research and understand experiences of nursing practice in the context of the nursing situation.

Sample

A purposive sample of eight participants was obtained from students enrolled in courses at a state university in southeastern United States. The criteria included being a registered nurse and currently practicing nursing.

Demographic data were obtained that included age, ethnicity, number of years in nursing, specialty area, highest earned degree and current program of study. The research participants were practicing registered nurses, age 22 years to 54 years of age with a median age of 39 years. Years in nursing ranged from 1.5 years to 33 years with a median of 18 years. Six participants were Caucasian, one was African-Caribbean and one was African-American. Highest earned degree data revealed six with a bachelor's degree in nursing, one had a master's degree in public health and one with an associate degree. The participants were all enrolled in a current program of study: six in masters track programs, one in a doctoral program and one in an RN-BSN program. Each participant had a unique practice specialty area: labor and delivery, neonatal intensive care, oncology, discharge/transitional care, community health, acute ortho-surgical, nursing education, and acute medical-surgical practice areas (See Appendix A). One potential limitation to the study is the current presence of all participants in an educational program. It is possible that their current study might predispose the participants to think more than other practicing nurses about philosophical issues.

Recruitment

Eight participants were recruited to be part of the sample through which to explore the question. After consents were signed, the researcher conducted interviews lasting up to one hour with each participant in a private room at the College of Nursing. The interviews were audio recorded with the expressed consent and permission of the participants, and an interview guide was followed (see Appendix B).

The researcher transcribed the audio tapes verbatim. For each interview, recording, and note taking instance, only an assigned number was used to identify the data. Field notes were recorded, general observations were made by the researcher during the interviews and audio recording. All notes, stories, identifying numbers, tape recordings, and transcripts were locked in the researcher's office and will be kept confidential in perpetuity.

Data Collection

The researcher utilized three recruitment strategies. The first was a 10-minute presentation to students in a classroom describing the study and informed consent process. The students were given the researcher's contact information if any wanted to inquire about the study in more detail or to volunteer to participate. Second, a recruitment flyer was posted at a prominent place in the student lunch room at the College of Nursing. The flyer included the study title and the researcher's email and phone number. Also, word of mouth was utilized to advertise the study and call for voluntary participants.

Research Question

What keeps nurses in nursing?

Interview Questions

Tell me a nursing situation about your best day in practice. There were follow up questions that may have helped clarify the participant's responses to the interview question (see Appendix B)

Data Analysis

Audio-taped interviews were transcribed verbatim by the researcher. The texts were read independently and interpretations of the data were compared and consensually validated by a member of the dissertation committee. The researcher conducted a hermeneutic analysis using Heideggerian hermeneutic phenomenology as the philosophical grounding to guide the identification of categories, relational themes and constitutive patterns of transcripts (Benner, Tanner & Chesla, 1996; Heidegger, 1927/1962). The intent was to describe meaning in the texts beyond the transcribed sentence as part of the larger whole and interpret the meaning from the context (Benner et al., 1996). The circularity of interpretation concerned the relation of parts to the whole and the interpretation of each part was dependent on the interpretation of the whole (Boykin & Schoenhofer, 2001).

Heideggerian hermeneutic phenomenology was the method for interpreting the phenomenon. Credibility of the data was established through dissertation committee member reviews and audit trails. Certain faculty members were selected to participate as peer reviewers as they are considered to be expert in interpretative phenomenology. They were chosen to review transcripts and verify consistent application of the method. Trustworthiness of the research data was established by the ability to trace information from the original source via an audit trail.

Based on the Heideggerian interpretive tradition, Dickleman and Allen (1989) described a seven-stage process of analysis of narrative texts. The stages are as follows:

Stage One

The data were transcribed and the transcripts were read as a whole to obtain an overall understanding of the texts.

Stage Two

Each transcript was reread and an individual summary was developed: 31 categories, units of meaning, were identified and a rich excerpt of the data was provided to support the category.

Stage Three

The transcripts were further evaluated and the categories were examined for similarities and differences among the groups.

Stage Four

Four relational themes were identified from the categories reflecting shared practice and common meanings.

Stage Five

The data were examined for emergence of a constitutive pattern that that linked all the themes and illuminated a shared meaning of the data.

Stage Six

The interpreted findings were reviewed, reflected upon and discussed with the dissertation committee members who were familiar with both the content and research method.

Stage Seven

The findings were prepared using sufficient excerpts from the transcripts for reader evaluation.

The multiple stages of interpretation provided a means for analyzing the data (Dickelman & Allen, 1989). Unfolding patterns were revealed in the transcribed texts as the participants told their story in the context of the nursing situation (Boykin & Schoenhofer, 2001; Newman, 1994, 2008).

The goal of hermeneutics is the discovery and understanding of meanings embedded in the text. Hermeneutics stems from systemic study of texts originally developed as a tool of biblical exegesis, jurisprudence, historical research and literary criticism (Benner, 1984; Polkinghorne, 1983). The process involves moving from the parts of the text, to the whole, and back to the parts again. Continuous examination of the whole and the parts of the transcripts with constant reference to the text ensured that interpretations were grounded and focused (Diekelmann & Allen, 1989).

The study design was exploratory and interpretive. The process of writing and rewriting was essential. The purpose of multiple levels of interpretations allowed for continuous participation and revealed contradiction and inconsistencies. The researcher described shared practices and common meanings until saturation and redundancy occurred (Diekelmann, & Allen, 1989).

Methodological Rigor

Strategies to ensure the accuracy of data collection and analysis were established using the framework described by Lincoln and Guba (1985) and elaborated by Sandelowski (1986). Lincoln and Guba (1985) describe rigor as trustworthiness and authenticity for qualitative methods and findings. Trustworthiness enabled qualitative inquiry to make a reasonable claim to methodological soundness and established rigor by using techniques that provide truth-value through credibility, applicability through transferability, consistency through dependability and neutrality through confirmability. Authenticity described the mechanism by which I ensured that the findings of the study were real, true and authentic (Lincoln & Guba, 1985). The four factors of trustworthiness to demonstrate scientific rigor as described by Lincoln and Guba (1985) are discussed below.

Credibility can be assured by spending time with the participants to control consistency, stability and repeatability of the analyses (Sandelowski, 1986). Prolonged engagement, which corroborates credibility and enhances trust with participants, was met by my years of experience as an RN. Interviews were intensive, open-ended and in-depth. Immersion in the data by myself and the dissertation committee constitutes representation of diverse experiences in nursing and anthropology, such as nursing leadership, nursing education, community nursing, surgical nursing, nursing history and medical anthropology. While prolonged engagement was provided scope, persistent observation did provide depth. Persistent observation involved the recruitment of nurses until saturation was achieved. Eight nurse participants volunteered to participate in the study. Lastly, I maintained a reflective journal that provided insight and aid in methodological decision making.

Transferability is described as judgments that will be facilitated through purposive and convenience sampling with inclusion of extensive quotations used in the analysis. The rich texts provided the information to judge the categories and themes sought by making the participants' stories and the findings valid, this was achieved by thoroughly capturing verbatim comments by the participants, immediate transcription of the tapes and detailed field notes.

Dependability was maximized using an audit trail that included maintaining a research journal in which both methodological decisions and the researcher's reactions and feelings were recorded. The reflective journal augmented the audit trail and help ensured confirmability.

Ethical Considerations

The investigator received approval from the Institutional Review Board of Florida Atlantic University. All participants' confidentiality was protected during the interviews. All notes, stories, identifying numbers, tape recordings and transcripts are kept under lock and key.

Once approval from the Institutional Review Board of Florida Atlantic University was obtained, I requested permission from faculty at the College of Nursing to present the study to nursing students in the classroom and to invite participation in this study. Using the informed consent process, participants were assured that their participation is voluntary and that they may withdraw at anytime without consequences. In appreciation of the participants' time, a Starbuck's Five Dollar Gift Card was given. Participants experienced minimal risks. The investigator was aware that the interview may trigger some emotional distress about their work. If this occurred, the investigator would terminate the interview and initiate support services. Another ethical consideration was the researcher's respectful approach. Voice matters and whatever dialogue occurred during the interview was listened to and respected. The use of silence as a technique encouraged thoughtful reflection on the nursing situation.

Heideggerian hermeneutic meaning in the text was derived from the lived experiences of nurses caring for their patient in the context of the nursing situation. The nurses' stories gave voice and vision to nurses' work and meaning. Nurses in practice are experts in the lived experience of nursing and meaning in their life-world and everydayness (Heidegger, 1927/1962). This method encouraged nurses to voice their experiences, thus emphasizing the importance of understanding the meaning of their experiences from their individual self-interpretive perspective while ethically respecting the voice of the expert nurses. Heideggerian hermeneutic phenomenology was the method to guide this research in order to discover and understand the nurses meaning that became embedded in the transcripts created from the audio recordings into rich text for analysis (Packer, 1989).

Chapter Summary

In this chapter, the qualitative research method of research and the phenomenological approach were described. The chapter also provided a description of the steps taken to obtain approval for the study, the plan for meeting potential participants, and the method for data collection, data analysis and interpretation. Additionally, methods to demonstrate scientific rigor, specifically trustworthiness and authenticity were delineated.

CHAPTER 4

FINDINGS

The findings presented in this chapter are descriptions of what "what keeps nurses in nursing" for the eight participants in this study. Heideggerian hermeneutical phenomenology philosophy and methodology provided the opening to understand this meaning of the human experience in nursing practice. Each participant's personal account, although unique, encompassed shared meanings and contributed to the overall understanding of the phenomenon. Each participant graciously offered the gift of presence and allowed the researcher to come to know each of them.

The data were analyzed utilizing Diekelmann and Allen's (1989) process for analysis of narrative texts utilizing the Heideggarian hermeneutical interpretative tradition (presented in Chapter 3). The analysis comprised the following seven stages:

Stage One

The data were transcribed and the transcripts were read as a whole to obtain an overall understanding of the texts.

Stage Two

Each transcript was reread and an individual summary was developed: 31 categories, units of meaning, were identified and a rich excerpt of the data was provided to support the category.

Stage Three

The transcripts were further evaluated and the categories were examined for similarities and differences among the groups.

Stage Four

Four relational themes were identified from the categories reflecting shared practice and common meanings.

Stage Five

The data were examined for emergence of a constitutive pattern that that linked all the themes and illuminated a shared meaning of the data.

Stage Six

The interpreted findings were reviewed, reflected upon and discussed with the dissertation committee members who were familiar with both the content and research method.

Stage Seven

The findings were prepared using sufficient excerpts from the transcripts for reader evaluation.

The data analysis is presented with an interpretive exemplar for each participant. The researcher identified 72 significant statements from the text. The researcher developed 31 supporting categories from the significant statements analysis. Then, four relational themes were synthesized from the supporting categories. Finally, the constitutive pattern that links the themes was identified. The interpretation of the data is fully described below.

Categories

The following data are provided using pseudonyms for the eight participants in this study. Each participant described multiple nursing situations to reflect their practice and expressed what keeps them in nursing. The synthesized descriptions below illustrate the fullness of each participant's nursing practice.

Participant #1: Mary

Mary is a 54-year-old woman, mother of two teenage daughters, who has been a registered nurse for 33 years. She was interviewed in a comfortable closed door well lit conference room. Mary was eager to share her nursing experience and explained that she has worked in one hospital her entire career, initially as a Labor and Delivery nurse. Then she became a case manager for 5 years. Presently she is the clinical nurse manager for Maternity, Newborn Services, Nursery, Labor and Delivery (L&D) and Neonatal Intensive Care Unit (NICU), and has been for the past 7 years. She is responsible for guiding the staff, doing interviews for hiring, providing annual evaluations, orientation, day to day scheduling and running of the unit. She reports that she provides consultation not only to the staff, but her patients and families as well. She makes sure that the patients are well cared for by the staff.

Mary states she started out in L&D and has enjoyed many good days being part of women experiencing the miracle of birth. No matter how many deliveries Mary has had the privilege to participate in she feels that "it is always a miracle." After 28 years of experience in delivering babies, she still appreciates the miracle of each birth and states, "No matter how many deliveries I see, it is always a miracle."

She stated "there were a lot of good days just being able to be part of women experiencing childbirth." After a long silent pause she declared "I have all these faces swirling in front of me…it's really hard to get it down to just one patient." "The best day in practice…wow, there have been so many of them."

She had difficulty deciding on one experience that really made a difference in the way she practices nursing, but finally offered the following story. The nursing situation involved a woman whom she had not met before. The women had delivered a non-viable fetus at 17 weeks gestation in the emergency department one week ago. After being home for a week the mother had decided she wanted to see the baby and to have a proper burial. The nursing supervisor was uncomfortable about making this happen for the mother and told Mary about the situation. Mary recounts noticing the supervisor's discomfort, Mary volunteers to help the women. Mary described that a non-viable fetus under 20 weeks gestation is sent to pathology and it is unusual to then plan for a burial. Mary went to the pathology department to get the baby; however, at this point, the baby is called the specimen. Mary found a baby's hat and clothes and she dressed the specimen. Mary assisted with the transition of the specimen to a baby after it was dressed and took the baby to the chapel for the mother to spend time with her baby.

> I said I'll do it; just find me a room, so we decided on the chapel in the hospital. Which I thought it was very appropriate as I met the mother with the baby, and it was just such a moving experience. I've never seen this

> woman before but I felt so close to her through this experience and afterwards and feel I really helped to make a difference in her bonding and grieving with her baby. We spent maybe an hour or an hour and a half together dressing the baby, taking pictures, arranging the baby with different items that she had and talking about it. I'd like to think that I made difference, you know, in her experience. It made it more of a positive experience for her.

In her present nursing position she states that "unfortunately I am not doing direct patient care, but I am called to the bedside when there is a problem: so now I still feel I can offer the patients a positive experience as much as possible." Mary's statement is interpreted as she is hoping that each Mother has the opportunity to take their baby home, "...I kind of just want that experience for all Mom's that they have a baby to take home."

Mary created the best situation possible so that a mother could grieve the loss of her 17-week-old fetus. Taking the baby from pathology as a specimen to be examined, she was able to creatively transition it to a baby boy by honoring the baby's babyhood. "I took the baby from the morgue, dressed him in a hat and gown and wrapped him in a blanket. I wanted it to look like a baby." She stated that the mother had an ultrasound picture with her and was told it was a boy, and declared "who am I to argue with that." Even when the baby was stillborn, Mary created the best situation for the baby and the mother, finding clothes, bringing them to the sacred place, the chapel, standing by, giving enough time for bonding, being present and capturing the experience with pictures.

The mother's call was to be able to bond with her baby boy. Mary was able to create the time and the space for the mother's to bond, even in her grief and bereavement, "I brought them to the chapel. This was her time with her baby." Mary made a difference "we took the time in her bonding, dressing the baby and taking pictures." She states that "I took my cue from her, I stepped back and did what she wanted me to, this was her time with her baby."

Mary declared that "I feel drawn to these types of experiences." She states she is aware that other nurses are not comfortable dealing with the death of a baby. She shares her compassion for the mother to be able to grieve in the best situation possible, "…end of a lot of dreams and hopes for her…need the time for Mom and baby." She also shares her compassion for her nurse colleagues who are not comfortable creating this caring encounter. Because of this experience Mary decided that she will obtain a certification in grief counseling in order to provide education for the staff and new nurses.

Mary hears the call to mentor new nurses. She desires to "create and provide an environment so new nurses can have a rewarding career as I have." She states "I would be supportive of her in making sure that she is connected with a good preceptor that it works out well." "To make sure it's a positive experience" to be able to energize the new nurse.

As one teaching example, Mary shared her passion by stating "when the new nurse is focused on the mother and baby breastfeeding successfully by taking the time needed, she experienced a very positive rewarding feeling, as well as the Mom and baby." The new nurse, mother and baby and Mary take the time intentionally to help the new mother learn to breast feed successfully.

Mary discussed that "everyone is born being able to care, that we learn it as we go through life and that it is being reinforced so that you know it's the right thing to do." She fulfills the needs of others and maintains a harmonious relationship and values "doing the right thing" in an ethical presence.

Eight categories emerged from the description of what is a best day at nursing practice for Mary and are presented with significant statements to support the category. A category table is presented to facilitate clarity.

Table 1

Category Development—Participant #1: Mary

Significant Statement	Category
"The best day in practice…wow, there have been so many of them."	Nursing is an evolving process of care
"No matter how many deliveries I see it is always a miracle"	Appreciating the miracle of each birth
"I was with a patient who had a fetal demise in the ER and I met her a week later. I kind of just want that experience for all Mother's that they have a baby to take home."	Hoping each Mother has a baby to take home or at least a memory of bonding.
"I took the baby from the morgue, dressed him in a hat and gown and wrapped him in a blanket. I wanted it to look like a baby."	Honoring the baby's babyhood.
"I brought them to the chapel. This was her time with her baby…"	Creating a sacred time and space for mother-baby bonding.
"I brought them to the chapel. This was her time with her baby…"	Creating a sacred time and space for mother-baby bonding.
	(Table continues)

Table 1 (*continues*)	
"End of a lot of dreams and hopes for her…need the time for Mom and baby"	Feeling the loss for mother and baby as compassion
"Mentoring new nurses so they can have a rewarding career that I had." I am geared toward clinical instruction…there is a need for nurses, so we need to get more students and nurses to make it a positive experience."	Energizing passion for nursing in new nurses.
"Caring is to be there for somebody, take care of the patient's whole situation. Everyone is born to care, we learn it as we go through life, it is being reinforced, you know that it's the right thing to do"	Caring as the ethical grounding in nursing

Participant #2: Winnie

Winnie is a 49-year-old woman who has been a registered nurse for 29 years. The last 18 of those years she has specialized as a Neonatal Intensive Care Unit (NICU) nurse, although she feels that her love for cardiac nursing has been a common thread throughout her entire career. She was interviewed in a quiet study room on the college campus to provide for confidentiality. Winnie expressed difficulty in coming up with a best day at practice by virtue of a long silent pause as she reflected on her nursing experiences. After reflecting she described a two year process of planning and implementing a complex life saving program, "…it took two years to set up the ECMO program." She stated, "I felt very proud when I accomplished that, it took a long time. We had to train therapists, the nurses, the perfusionists and physicians and do the education in the lab and even the animal lab." She continued, "Some hospitals put perfusionists at the bedside, so I am very proud that we're putting nurses to run the pump because I felt that they would look at the babies differently than the perfusionist at the bedside." Winnie stated she "really enjoyed setting up the ECMO program" as she finds joy in her practice in developing a complex technical program

The nursing situation she began to describe came from her being chosen by hospital administration to plan, set up and implement the ECMO (extra corporal membrane oxygenation) program in her hospital. This program was the first in the county. ECMO is temporary support of heart and lung function by partial cardiopulmonary bypass. It is used for neonates who have reversible cardiopulmonary failure from pulmonary, cardiac or other disease. Blood is drained from the neonate to an external pump which pushes the blood through a membrane gas exchanger for oxygenation and carbon dioxide removal. The blood circulates through a warmer and is returned to the neonate's circulation. Winnie stated that there was a dire need for this program to save babies lives at the hospital of their birth and preventing long transportation to another facility, during which, the baby was at risk. She explained that treating the babies where they were born prevented unnecessary travel on the road to seek this life saving service.

Winnie described a nursing situation with a mother who wanted her baby to be the first to have this life saving treatment. The baby suffered many set backs and subsequently the parents decided that this life saving measure should be discontinued. Winnie described how she felt torn between caring for the baby and the mother with technology and then with bereavement support. It became important for Winnie to have the mother hold her baby for the first time while he was still alive, stating that the mother had never had the chance to hold her baby. Winnie needed to continue the ECMO pump while assisting the mother to hold her baby for the first time. Winnie knew that as soon as the pump was shut off, the baby would die. It was important for the mother to hold her baby for the first and last time.

> …when we opened the baby up, to do surgery on the heart-lung bypass, all the intestines were like dark black with horrible perfusion. So I watched the surgery, and I just was like 'oh my,' you know, how are we going to salvage that gut because every loop of bowel that the surgeon brought out was black and the baby was in shock a long time. I

came to work on the night shift just to fill-in and the baby was black from the waist down. The baby was less than 3 weeks old actually by then, we were less than three weeks on ECMO, which is a really long time, but the baby was completely black and mottled from the waist down. We had the ECMO machine that was keeping the baby alive. But then, it was mechanically like we were just keeping the baby alive, but the baby, was, you know… how can you be from your waist down totally black without perfusion, crunchy, you know, gangrenous looking thing. And I came on, and I just looked at the baby and looked at the mom and I looked at the director, and it was just like, you know, what are we doing here? The longer you are on the pump the more complications there are. We had a lot of hope for the baby, he was a big chubby, you know, it wasn't like a premature baby. He was a term baby, and had a diaphragmatic, congenital diaphragmatic hernia. They do the worst statistically on the heart-lung machine. Mom wanted to be the first and she knew she had that kind of baby and she knew we would possibly put the baby on the machine and she was glad and she was happy to be able to do it and so, it was upsetting, because it was the beginning of the program, but we talked to the mom, and we decided to stop the pump. I wanted to let her hold the baby and be on the heart lung bypass machine, which is very dangerous

> scary thing, as you have a cannula going into the aorta and you know, there's all this blood and all the equipment, and it's just a big production to even get an x-ray, or turn them a little bit. So, I maneuvered everything, I wanted her to hold the baby while the baby was still alive, she had never held the baby.

She had a lot of hope for the first baby that was a candidate for ECMO, "the baby had a congenital diaphragmatic hernia and they do the worst statistically on the machine." The parents decided that it was time to take the baby off the machine. Before that was to happen, Winnie made sure that the mother held the baby for the first time while the baby was still alive, "…she never held the baby, her baby, ever." The mother had never held her baby, and Winnie had the compassion to make it happen for the mother, feeling the feeling of the other. By thinking ahead, she thought it would help the mother with bereavement and to have some time with the baby while still alive on the machine.

Winnie spoke of some of her families and exclaimed, "I really like the family-centered care, and I like treating the whole family", expressing openness and wholeness in the nursing situation. Winnie experienced a commitment to the ECMO program, "I had been there every day, I was there every single day. I was calling in to check on things. I had been on call for two years and never gotten called in." She devoted herself to the program with willingness and commitment.

Winnie described the fear and how scared the staff was in training and then actually performing this highly technical complex care, "we were scared and excited, it's very dangerous and stressful for the person learning and for the parent." She discovered through her experience that she had the courage to make hope possible.

Winnie stated that she will be going to a birthday party for one of her babies; he will be 4 or 5 years old. She stays connected and goes to his birthday party every year. At the party the family introduces her as the person who saved the baby's life. The family played a video of his hospitalization when he got the Last Rites. The video was uplifting because at the end the baby went home with the red carpet and roses.

During the baby's hospitalization the OR tech had insisted that the baby and nurse take the usual path to the operating room. Winnie disagreed and insisted they take the long way around. On the long way to the OR, they were able to stop where the whole entire family waited and prayed over the isolette, "I had to fight to do it but then he saw it really was the right thing when he saw what I was doing." The OR tech cried and she stated that he realized that this was the right thing to do and thanked Winnie for the loving spiritual experience. Winnie guided ethical caring in a complex nursing situation.

Winnie described how she always thinks ahead. Being family centered with an ongoing presence, "I stay connected a while until I feel they are OK." She described the nature of her nursing as ethical caring in a complex environment and created the best nursing situation possible, "…constantly scanning the environment to see if your little ecosystem is providing enough humidity, does the skin look good, is there any breakdown… constantly scanning the environment to see what's the best thing.".

Ten categories emerged from the description of what is a best day at nursing practice for Winnie and are presented with significant statements to support the category. A table is presented to facilitate clarity.

Table 2

Category Development—Participant #2: Winnie

Significant Statement	Category
A long silent pause…reflecting on her nursing experiences; "…it took two years to set up the ECMO program."	Expressing one experience in a best day of practice was difficult; nursing is an evolving process
"I really enjoyed setting up the ECMO program…it was the first ECMO center in the county to put babies on the	Finding joy in her practice in developing a complex technical program to care (*table continues)*
Table 2 (*continued*)	
heart-lung machine." "I felt	for each family member

very proud that we were putting nurses to run the pump"	
"I really like the family centered care, and I like treating the whole family."	Opening the nursing situation with wholeness
"It was big and chubby…it was a term baby, it had a congenital diaphragmatic hernia and they do the worst statistically on the machine." "Mom wanted to be the first, she knew she had that kind of baby and she would possible put the baby on the machine …and she was happy to be able to do it."	Hoping that the baby would grow with possibilities
"I wanted her to hold the baby while the baby was still alive, she never held the baby, her baby, ever."	Feeling the feeling of the other, compassion (thinking ahead, to hold the baby)
"I had been there everyday, I was there every single day, I was calling in to check on things. I had been on call for two years and never gotten called in."	Devoting self by commitment to the program
"I had been there everyday, I was there every single day, I	Devoting self by commitment *(table continues)*

Table 2 (*continues*)

was calling in to check on	to the program.

things. I had been on call for two years and never gotten called in."	
"We were scared, we were excited. It's very dangerous so, it's very stressful for the person learning it and it's also very scary for the parent."	Experiencing courage to make hope possible
"I stay connected a while until I feel they are OK"	Ongoing presence to provide an environment for healing
"…I had to fight to do it but then he saw it was really the right thing when he saw what I was doing." "To make sure all my T's are crossed and my I's are dotted and I am moving in the right way…where you expect them to be, and if not you herd them, like a shepherd."	Guiding ethical care in a complex situation
.".constantly scanning the environment to see if your little ecosystem is providing enough humidity, does the skin look, is there any breakdown… constantly scanning the environment to see what's the best thing."	Caring for person and environment to create the best situation

Participant #3: Fran

Fran is a 49-year-old woman who has been a registered nurse for 28 years, her specialty is hematology-oncology nursing. She has been a clinical educator for the past 6 years and is attending graduate school in the education track. She was interviewed in a quiet comfortable well lit conference room.

> Last week I had a patient; her husband had a really abrasive personality. She had ovarian cancer, and she was very thin and frail, she came to the hospital for her chemotherapy. Her husband is the kind of man that will takeover and act like "I'll speak for you," and "I'll do for you, and you just sit back and I'll take care of everything." He was yelling at the nursing staff, and he just was very abrasive and she was having difficulty with her chemotherapy. She was starting to get a little confused, and he was just beside himself, he was just beside himself. I had already made a connection with him because he was frustrated with the nursing staff before, and I was there and I made that special connection with him and reassured him that we were going to meet her needs and by meeting her needs, we were meeting his. She was really having a tough afternoon and she couldn't seem to calm herself down, she was just really anxious and he was looking to me like what's wrong with her, what's wrong with her, she was very anxious and she was hallucinating, but she was just so anxious. I put her up

> against my chest and I put her head on my chest and I was rubbing her back, and I was just stroking her and telling her that she was going to be okay and that everything was going to be okay and this went on for 15 to 20 minutes. In the meantime, I was on the phone and I called her nurse and asked her to bring some Xanax. The nurse medicated her with Xanax and then I put the lights off and turned off the TV and kept holding and rubbing her until she finally relaxed a little bit and she lay back in the bed and she went to sleep. It was interesting because the next day I went to visit her to see how she was doing and she was just as she sat up straight in that bed and said "AHH , you're here!" Even though she was so confused a day before, I never expected her to remember that, I never did, but she did and she totally remembered that. I had held her in my arms, and I had rubbed her back and she remembered that comforting. It was wonderful experience. Nurturing a patient like that that is really very satisfying.

Fran had difficulty deciding on one experience that really made a difference in the way she practices nursing. She stated, "my role is varied…it would just be a usual day at work visiting with patients."

Fran stated that her usual day at practice consisted of visiting patients in her role of educator. She makes it a point to see patients with sickle cell anemia on her floor. She states that "they are just such a pleasure, but are not always kind people…because of their pain." Fran continued explaining that she has a love for all her patients who have sickle cell anemia.

Fran stated that it is painful to see a patient in pain and described a feeling of being helpless. Fran makes it a point to visit patients who return due to suffering from sickle cell anemia. One particular patient had child care problem at home and Fran was able to mobilize family resources so that the young daughter would be safe. On a previous admission, Fran gave the patient a special crocheted blanket. The patient told her that her daughter "takes that special blanket everywhere." She described this nursing situation as "really very satisfying." She stated that she realized she is "in the right place, at the right time, doing the right thing. I just know that I am doing God's work." Fran experienced a spiritual call as being called to the wholeness of nursing practice.

Fran gave the description of a patient weeping after being diagnosed with cancer and asks rhetorically "what do you say?" She knows that what came out of her is the Holy Spirit that reached out to the patient. She continued to say "I mean, there are so many times when my skills couldn't really do what needs to be done, even a simple thing like starting an IV. There's no vein there, there's absolutely no vein and you put the needle in and you let the Holy Spirit find whatever is there. It's not me." Fran describes practicing nursing as spiritual care.

Fran described reflecting on nursing situations in which she had felt satisfaction as she responded to the nursing call uniquely, "Sometimes I have the time to reflect on that feeling right away, I get a real personal high and sometimes I am too attuned into the clinical situation.." She stated it takes time, time to intentionally do the personal reflection and to take the time to think. When she experienced the personal high as joy, she described it as an "adrenalin rush" that is energizing.

Fran intentionally created space for a caring presence as a way of being that allowed awareness for nurse and patient to connect. She created time and space for a caring presence when, "my very first nurse manager took me by the hand and said, all the bronchodilators, all the respiratory treatments will not help the patients the way your presence will, then she sat me down and showed me how sitting with a patient and pursed lip breathing with him will calm the patient down much better than any medication. This was my introduction to presence." Fran described how her mentors helped her to come to know herself in a caring relationship.

Fran expressed that being satisfied in nursing for her is that "I touched somebody in a special way…to be in the right place at the right time and doing the right thing." For Fran it is important to know that she made a difference in somebody's life by doing the right thing as ethical caring.

Ten categories emerged from the description of what is a best day at nursing practice for Fran and are presented with significant statements to support the category. A table is presented to facilitate clarity.

Table 3

Category Development—Participant #3: Fran

Significant Statements	**Category**
"My role is very varied…it would just be a usual day at work visiting with patients"	Nursing is an evolving process of care
"I just know that I am doing God's work. I know that this is what God has planned for me."	Being called to the wholeness of nursing practice
"When a patient is weeping because they have just been told they have cancer, what do you say? …I'm just, whatever comes out of me. I truly believe it's the Holy Spirit coming through."	Responding uniquely in the moment to calls for nursing
"Even simple thing like starting an IV, there's no vein there. There is absolutely no vein, and you just put the needle in and you let the holy Spirit find whatever is there, and it's not me."	Practicing nursing as spiritual care (*table continues*)

<u>Table 3 (*continues*)</u>	
"Sometimes I have the time to reflect on that feeling right away and then sometimes I get a real personal high and sometimes I am too attuned into the clinical situation."	Reflecting on practice
"The personal high feels like an adrenalin rush..."	Experiencing joy as a personal high that is energizing
"I think I have had, always have had nurse leaders and nurse mentors, who kind of mentored me in this type of role and this type of relationship."	Mentoring in a caring relationship
"My very first nurse manager took me by the hand and said, all the bronchodilators, all the reparatory treatments will not help the patients the way your presence will, then she sat me down and showed me how sitting with a patient and pursed lip breathing with him will calm the patient down much better than any medication. This was my introduction to presence."	Learning how to create time and space for a caring presence
"I have always been the nurse on the floor that would be the preceptor or the nurse to explain	Knowing self (*table continues*)

Table 3 (*continues*) things. That's just who I am, it comes naturally"	
"Being satisfied in nursing, I know that it is for me that I touched somebody in a special way…to be in the right place at the right time, doing the right thing"	Making a difference in ethical caring.

Participant #4: Marie

Marie is a 28-year-woman who has been a registered nurse for five and a half years. Initially she worked nights on a medical-surgical floor. Presently she is working at the newly formed discharge courtesy lounge at the same hospital where she has been working since graduation from nursing school. She states she has experienced many good days nursing.

> My best day nursing, oh, there's been many of them. But one day recently I was having one of those personal cruddy days, when you just don't want to get out of bed, don't want to go to work, and wondered why I became a nurse, type of days. And there was this very nice woman, who had open heart surgery. Where I work right now, I discharge people home. I basically take their entire chart and make sure that all the discharge planning and proper education gets done

> before they leave the hospital. I think I spent a good hour and a half with her, just going over everything from her diabetes, postop course, everything for her safe discharge home. I know we had a difficult time getting her in the car because she was a very large woman and she had the surgery and chest incision that we couldn't get the seat belt around her properly. We had to move her to the back seat. So by the time I was done, I was like, this is why I am a nurse because anyone else might had just rolled her outside and said, good luck. It just made me feel good when I was done. That I helped her and she was going home safely and she had a smile on her face when she was leaving the hospital.

Marie continued describing her rewarding nursing career and that helping people is the reason she chooses to stay in nursing. She stated that helping people makes her feel good and describes the good feeling as satisfaction, a "warm and fuzzy" euphoric feeling. She states that when she has the good feeling, she knows that she has done the right thing and declares "it's doing the right thing for the patient."

Marie states that she has had so many best days in her nursing practice. She eagerly gave multiple examples of how she has made a difference in her patient's lives. Marie shared, "I have the knowledge to help people, and people trust us as nurses also, they trust me with their personal information. That's one thing that helps me to continue to be a nurse, that I help people."

Marie stated that it is important to her to make a difference. When asked how she experienced making a difference she laughed and said, "it makes you come back the next day" and that she felt energized by caring. She explained that she gets a sense of gratification helping her patients and she thinks it is rewarding to help people. Over time and with experience she felt that she knew a little bit more and she was able to get the benefits from the job.

She described that what keeps her in nursing is the satisfied feeling that she intentionally helped somebody. She asserts "my hope is that I helped them and then I am satisfied you know that I've made a difference…did the right thing for the patient. It gave me a sense of satisfaction that I did the right thing for the patient that I cared for the entire patient, not just his medical needs."

Marie stated that she has gained confidence and competence over time. She described that she has been able to spend more time being with her patients and stated, "and now I know what I am doing a little bit more, I'm able to get the benefits of the job."

Marie explains that she enjoys working with her fellow nurses and states, "we are the example of team work." She described a culture of caring for each other and taking care of each other.

Marie explained that her nurse colleagues will discuss the negative aspects of the job to let it out. She declares that it is important to share the "good stuff" and not simply just hold onto the positive feelings, to celebrate the joy of nursing.

Marie experienced compassion as an internal motivation to do good and the right thing as valuing and respect for the other. She described a situation when discharging a homeless patient, it was not important to find a home, but it was important to discharge him to get safely to whatever the patient considered home. In so doing she respected the patient and valued the whole person as well as the person's environment. She declared "I may not make a difference in everybody's life but at least once a day, I make a difference in somebody's life."

Eight categories emerged from the description of what is a best day at nursing practice for Marie and are presented with significant statements to support the category. A table is presented to facilitate clarity.

Table 4

Category Development—Participant #4: Marie

Significant Statements	Category
"There have been so many of them."	Nursing is an evolving process of care
"Why did I become a nurse....by the time I was done, this was why I am a nurse." "You know that you have made a difference, it makes you come back the next day."	Being energized by caring
"...my hope that I helped them and then I am satisfied you know you've made a difference...did the right thing for the patient. It gave me a sense of satisfaction that I did the right thing for the patient that I cared for the entire patient, not just his medical needs."	Doing the right thing intentionally
"And now I know what I am doing a little bit more, I'm able to get the benefits of the job."	Gaining confidence and competence to be able to spend more time being with the patient
'We work as a team and take care of each other...there is a culture of caring, definitely, we are an example of teamwork."	Caring for fellow nurses, collegiality and team work

(*table continues*)

Table 4 (*continues*)	
"…if they're homeless then its not important for them to find a home…but it is important for them to get safely to whatever they consider home."	Valuing and respect for the whole person and environment
"I may not make a difference in everybody's life, but at least once a day I make a difference in somebody's life."	Making a difference
"…hold on to the positive feelings and talk about the negative stuff, just let it out. We should share to good stuff too"	Celebrating the joy of nursing

Participant #5: Sue

Sue is a 52-year-old woman who has been a registered nurse for 30 years and has a master's degree in public health. She has worked with children who have chronic illnesses and their families for 18 years. For the past 2 years she has been a case manager in a community hospital caring for children who have sustained traumatic brain injuries.

> I really do have to think about it because I've been doing this for long, I mean, there is so much. I don't know why and this goes way back frankly to when I was a nursing

> student but it's probably part of what touched me in nursing and kept me in nursing. It's actually a fairly depressing story but I remember as a nursing student the first patient I took care of who died while I was kind of the primary nursing student involved. I remember his name; I remember his family. He was a relatively young man who had leukemia. This was probably thirty years ago when people did not necessary survive with leukemia as they do now. And I remember being so frightened as a nursing student about what was happening and what his care needs were. I remember how gracious he and his family were in receiving care. I just remembered being so kind of touched by that. That situation really spoke to me about what was the dual process; that it really is a nurse/patient relationship or a patient/nurse relationship or a person/person relationship. That made a huge impression on me, so much so that when you asked me about a good day in nursing, I go back to it and that was a long time ago and a different experience ago because that was in acute care and I haven't worked in acute care for many, many, many years. .

She described her experiencing nursing as an evolving process over the past 30 years, "I really do have to think about it because I've been doing this so long, I mean, there is so much." Sue stated that "people bring a grace with them when they are not feeling well or are impacted by a health issue. Recognizing the patient's grace is important as it is where you meet the person." Sue describes this "grace" as coming to know the other and coming to understand the other from within. Finding the grace in the other is the beginning of the caring relationship. Sue explained that it is the patient relationship that is satisfying for her in nursing. She further stated that it is respect first and foremost. "I don't think that you can nurse, I don't think you can intervene, I don't think you can help, I don't think you can do anything, unless you have a relationship."

Sue continued to describe how she has come to know self as nurse to be able to make a difference with presence, "at the end of the day I feel good about who I am and what I do. I feel as though my life and my presence and my being there, I make a difference in a good way, it validated what I do."

Sue described that she makes a positive difference in people's lives because of who she is. "It's not just the knowledge; it's not just the information. It's presence." When asked what she thought kept her in nursing she replied, "Well, I would like to tell you that it's something novel, but it's inertia in a positive way in that I've really enjoyed what I've been doing." She continued to explain inertia as a comfort zone that she is comfortable doing what she does. It is a comfortable state for her to work in and continually keeps her moving forward.

The good of what the nurse is doing keeps her going and is experienced as energy. Nursing presence keeps the nurse in nursing, doing something of value, to give back, is meaningful for the nurse, "making the world a better place one person at a time, healing the world." What the nurse brings to the patients' life is who the nurse is and she makes the difference, this validates who the nurse is and what the nurse does, and it is grounding. The patient's grace (call) is where the nurse meets the patient to answer the call as the nurse makes herself available as the call-to-care. Sue sends out the call to her patient by making the relationship a nurturing and caring place (Lesniak, 2008).

Six categories emerged from the description of what is a best day at nursing practice for Sue and are presented with significant statements to support the category. A table is presented to facilitate clarity.

Table 5

Category Development—Participant #5: Sue

Significant Statements	***Category***
"I really do have to think about it because I've been doing this long, I mean, there is so much."	Nursing evolving as a process of care.
'There is a grace people bring when they are not feeling well and when they have been impacted by a health issue. It's it is the part where you meet the person."	Finding grace in the other as the beginning of the caring relationship
"At the end of the day I feel good about who I am, I feel good about what I do. I feel as though my life and my presence and my being here makes a difference in a good way. Validates what I do."	Making a difference and presence; Knowing self
"I think it comes from respecting first and foremost, before a relationship has to be established.'	Respecting for other
"…inertia in a positive way which is as long as I've really enjoyed what I have been doing."	Moving forward from a point of inertia: the grounding of a thoughtful practice

(*table continues*)

Table 5 (*continues*)	
"…it's feeling that I am doing something of value. Giving back, making the world a better place one person at a time, healing the world."	Valuing what I do in making the world a better place

Participant #6: Amy

Amy is a 25-year-old woman working on an orthopedic and surgical floor for one and one half years. This is her first nursing job after obtaining her associate's degree and she currently is enrolled in a RN to BSN program. She recalls a good day nursing as one in which the unit was very organized and the work flowed well because of the charge nurse. She expressed that she enjoyed working as a team and appreciates the support and resources of her nurse expert colleagues.

Amy described a recent patient she cared for who had experienced the death of her baby. She recalled that her patient was grieving over the loss of her second child. Amy stated, "You know, I'm a woman too and I knew just how heartbroken she must have felt in losing her child. Helping her sort of made me realize why I am in nursing and what I can do to help people transition back home." It was a sad experience, but Amy did take time for herself to think about her patient situation. She stated that she is spiritual so in this situation that made her feel overwhelmed, she needed to take a minute to nurse herself, by having a conversation with the Lord. The patient was her first maternity patient and she went to her charge nurse for support and to be able to express her feelings of sadness, compassion and wanting to cry.

> Okay, I have one. I had the chance to stick with my patient and explain with the doctor present what was going on with her body even though this wasn't her first miscarriage, it was the first time she understood what had happened. I remember after that experience I sort of made a personal decision that I would make time for that one-to-one interaction to actually nurse my patient. I remember when I had to I went into her room just to say my goodbye and she just held my hand and gave me a big hug and said thank you so much for just explaining and taking the time, that I really cared. I won't forget that interaction and I try to make that kind of interaction everyday when I go to work. I'm a woman too and I could see just how heartbroken she was and I felt broken hearted too. I remember helping her at that moment and it made me realize that I am in nursing and what I can do is to help people transition from the hospital back to their lives at home. I was sad and hurting for her, it was like a blended feeling. I did take a minute to myself, to collect myself but the day continues. You have other patients to tend to, but it did make that moment

helpful to think about it for a little bit. I'm spiritual so, situations that overwhelmed me, I just have to take a minute to sort of nurse myself. So I just felt the need to take a minute to have a conversation with the Lord. I'm more of a bubbly personality person and smiling and you know going in the room with patients saying "good morning." But it's like the moment I look in that door you can just sense that if I go in there and say "good morning" it is just inappropriate. So at that entire time I wasn't quite as perky because of her situation and how it touched me. I saw just how she was, you know you grieve for a loss and you slowly regain back to your life and she had family and friends to call her and told her things were going to get better. So as she sort of recovered from this I thought she was heading towards a healthy path of getting over that loss. By the end of the shift I wasn't sad any more. I think she touched my heart with the interactions that we had but I went home and went back to life. I don't think I remembered her until you asked me to talk about a good day nursing. I saw nursing as more than just task oriented. I could actually be a nurse in nursing the patient and o more than just doing dressings and passing out medications. I have certain patients who touch me and with her it was just… as the day went on and saying how she was talking on the phone with her family and things and she was

> getting up and doing her care and eating her lunch with encouragement, she didn't touch her breakfast. She was getting up and eating a little bit more. By dinner she was saying she was hungry so the trays came. It was nice to see that and so I felt even though she's a patient, I felt like I took the time to nurse myself as I was hurting because of her situation that touched me. So by the end of the day I just felt like things were moving as they should and she was progressing through a grief process and was getting back to herself. I went to my charge nurse and other colleagues to sort of express my feelings and they also sort of responded that it's going to be okay. You know, you have patients that will touch you. I think you can over sympathize with patients but you know, I do think it is okay to have that feeling because you're human yourself and people go through situations which are painful and sad. But, you know, I could one day go through it myself and so you put yourself in their shoes.

Amy was quick to describe an experience when she had a best day nursing. She described an entire shift, rather than a specific nursing situation. Amy spoke of her charge nurse being responsible for the flow on the unit and stated that the medication computer system was functioning, the patients were getting better and even the doctors were cooperating. She described the whole atmosphere as an evolving process of care.

Amy described the experience of caring for a mother who had lost her second baby. Amy stated that she was hurting for the mother and had the opportunity to be with her when the doctor came to explain what had happened to her body. This was not the patients' first loss, but it was the first time the patient understood what had happened. Amy remembered the experience and made a conscious decision that, in the future, she would make time for a one-to-one interaction with each patient in order to actually nurse her patients. Amy expressed how she was feeling compassion, "I was hurting for her. She touched my heart with the interaction we had."

Amy described how she took the time to nurse herself by praying to the Lord as she felt sad and hurt for the mother. She stated "I did take a minute to myself to collect myself but the day continued and I had other patients to tend to. It changed how I saw nursing to be more than just task oriented. I could do more than just do dressing changes and passing out medications. I could actually be a nurse to nurse the patient."

Amy described herself as spiritual, when a situation overwhelmed her, she took the time to nurse herself. She had come to know that she is at the bedside for a purpose. She stated, "It's part of my job to make sure the patient's comfort needs are met." Amy described how she was comforting her patient with intention. Caring for her patients gives her a sense of worth. "When I make a patient comfortable, she or he is not in pain and then, she or he can enjoy the day that much better."

Amy explains how she experiences the patient as whole with a life outside of the hospital, "people who are in the hospital for a reason, they have a life outside the hospital and that I am nursing them and what I can do to help people transition."

Amy intentionally nurses with a purpose as she described how she gets to know her patient on an intimate level to make the interaction both important and significant. She stated, "Just to know that you are there for a purpose, you have a purpose, a reason to be there…it could be simply doing God's work." Amy is spiritually guided to do the work of nursing and the work of God.

Amy described caring-for-self by asking for help, and by asking for help, she honors the other. She is building trust in an intimate relationship with caring other purposefully that is validating and rewarding. She called it "a sense of worth." She illuminated self-worth in the dwelling place called nursing. Amy experienced nursing spiritually with purpose. Compassion is felt for the patient and self. Amy experienced caring with positive reinforcement as a "boost of energy." She described how she makes a difference intentionally by, "I try to make a difference one-be-one, little by little, I love having 12 hours to make that difference in care."

Nine categories emerged from the description of what is a best day at nursing practice for Amy and are presented with significant statements to support the category. A table is presented to facilitate clarity.

Table 6

Category Development—Participant #6: Amy

Significant Statements	**Category**
"…seemed like everyone flows and even our patients were better, it was the whole atmosphere."	Nursing is an evolving process of care
"I was hurting for her. She touched my heart with the interaction we had."	Feeling compassion
"It's part of my job to make sure that their comfort needs are met."	Comforting intentionally
"…people who are in the hospital for a reason that they have a life outside of the hospital that I am nursing and what I can do to help people transition."	Seeing the patient as a whole with a life outside of the hospital
"Like you are there for a purpose, to be there to nurse them…"	Nursing with a purpose
	(*table continues*)

Table 6 (*continues*)	
"…just to know that you are there for a purpose, you have a purpose, reason to be there…it could be just simply doing God's work."	Doing God's work
"I get a sense of worth. It's more like internal."	Doing something of value, reciprocal
"it gives me a boost of energy which always makes me feel good."	Being energized by nursing
"I make that difference and I try to make that difference one-by-one, little by little, I love having 12 hours to make that difference in care."	Making a difference intentionally

Participant #7: Ann

Ann is a 27-year-old woman who has been a registered nurse for 6 years. She currently is in the academic program chair for patient care technician students. When asked about her best day nursing, she had difficulty as she stated she has had so many experiences. After taking some quiet time to reflect, she chose a nursing situation from her pediatric experience.

> There are so many things to explore, you know, you're not isolated and you're not fixated in one spot. So, that's the

thing I love about nursing is the flexibility and the specialties, there are so many specialties you know. I have been a nurse for 6 years but I've worked in different areas. I'm trying to think of a pediatrics scenario that I had, a lot of them are sad though. I'm trying to think…pediatrics… what happened. Oh, gosh. Okay, my best day I would say was when I was taking care of a patient and I think it was a month old, and I was by myself. I had just moved from an acute care area and I got my pediatric floor orientation, so I was pretty confident in what I was doing. I had nursed adult care the year before so, I was a bit more experienced than the brand new nurses. I had a baby that I was feeding and, I know I laugh now in hindsight but, the baby stopped breathing and I was just like… I kind of paused for a minute but instinctively I just grabbed the Ambu bag and just, you know, was able to revive the baby and have the baby breathing again and I just remember in that moment that fear I felt and that I was able to move, able to do something. That was the very first time it happened to me. I think that was a memorable day for me because in that moment I realized that this is what makes the difference you know, being able to do that and being able to help with life and bring life back and sustain life. I felt it was energy promoting because it was in me, a defining moment for me. It let me know that I could actually do this. Actually, experiencing that and that I was able to act quickly, I knew that in a moment at any other time it could happen and I was confident and that was high energy for me. In school I learned all these things and never actually had a chance to do it. So for me it just made the difference of why I became a nurse. That was important to me to be able to rescue the baby. That was very important to me. That made me feel great because I was confident in what I knew and my ability, my skills, and the knowledge and the time that I spent in school. A lot of times when you're in school and its all theory and then when you get into steady work you're afraid because you ask, 'am I going to remember everything; am I going to do this right; is a patient going to perish because I don't know what I'm doing'. So in that moment it really gave me assurance that I know what I am doing, I was able to compose myself and act quickly. It reaffirmed why I'm in nursing and why I was able to help somebody and to make a difference in their life you know because I've seen a lot of people not act properly or as responsibly. I think some people have characteristics that they really need to be trained in a certain way. They need to train their mind to be detail oriented or disciplined and some people don't have that necessarily. They've gone into nursing and they just know the theory but there is some discipline that goes along with it as well. Nurses should be

> determined. I think that takes training. My issue is working along side people that I feel are inadequate because they do not put forth the same type of energy. The energy I put forth. I fine-tooth-comb my charts, my orders, recheck things assess and reassess my patients head to toe. Some people want to get out of work on time, so things are not done completely, they miss medications, they skip dressing changes, to me it's a scary thing. Its required energy, if you want to be effective and efficient, then high energy is required. The only thing that is going to produce those results is having high energy, positive energy to be caring and understanding while multitasking.

Ann was asked about a nursing situation when she had her best day nursing. She replied with a giggle, "my best day, wow, so many experiences. I have got to think…" She described how she has worked in many different areas and was trying to recall when she worked with a pediatric patient, she had a difficult time deciding on a nursing situation.

Ann stated that as a nurse with confidence, it reaffirms why she is in nursing, has the ability to help somebody, and make a difference. She continues "you know, I've seen a lot of people not act properly or responsibly. I think some people need to be trained in certain ways, they need to train their mind to be detailed oriented or disciplined." She described being disciplined as an exposure to experiences in order to learn to be more detail oriented, to be prepared and ready for anything.

Ann stated that by being competent "I belong there, I should be there, I have the skills and ability to be there." She stated that she has a feeling of belonging and being in the right place. Ann explained that she doesn't work on the floor any longer because she has an issue working alongside people whom she feels are inadequate to the tasks and do not put forth required energy . "If you want to be effective, you have to be efficient, that's what is required." She described how she holds her own values by doing the right thing as an ethical stance. Ann declared that "I can't be apathetic, that's the energy training piece." Nursing is energizing and that is how Ann makes a difference for her patients.

Ann described that building confidence assists her to adapt to any situation and moves her nursing forward. It is important to pay attention to details so you can make a difference to the patient in need and this is energy promoting for the nurse. Confidence building is an energy promoting factor, creative energy is drawn from experience to express knowledge. She spoke about the pediatric nursing situation when a one month old she was feeding stopped breathing and she knew what to do. Ann was confident and created the nursing situation with competence.

Ann declares that a nurse will not receive tangible words, "Nobody's going to say 'here's notice for doing such a great job' and you rarely hear the thank you because it is expected, it's your job, it's your profession." She feels the reciprocity inwardly and doesn't need to be thanked.

Nine categories emerged from the description of what is a best day at nursing practice for Ann and are presented with significant statements to support the category. A table is presented to facilitate clarity.

Table 7

Category Development—Participant #7: Ann

Significant Statements	Category
"Wow, so many experiences, I have got to think about it."	Nursing is an evolving process of care
"…the opportunities in nursing keep me going…there are many things to explore."	Delighting in the many opportunities
"I realize that this is what makes the difference you know, being able to do that and being able to help with life and bring back life and sustain life. So for me it just made the difference of you know why I became a nurse."	Making a difference
"… to be more detailed oriented with the babies especially while feeding them and being prepared, have the ambu by your side that the equipment to use can give you the feeling of making a difference."	Creating the situation with competency
"I'm competent and I belong here, I have the skills and ability to be there."	Feeling of belonging, being in the right place
"My issue is working alongside people that are I feel are…inadequate…they don't put forth the same type of energy."	Holding with her own values
"have to have energy to get things done right, high energy is required."	Doing the right thing,

(*table continues*)

Table 7(*continues*)	an ethical stance
"…and then you rarely hear the thank you because it's your job, it's your profession."	Feeling the reciprocity inwardly, doesn't need to be thanked
"I can't be apathetic, that's the energy training piece"	Nursing is energizing

Participant #8: Beth

Beth is a 31-year-old woman who continues in her first nursing job of 10 years, and most recently she has accepted the charge nurse position. When asked about a time she experienced her best day nursing, she recalled a nursing situation at the beginning of her nursing career.

> Actually, the beginning of my nursing career when I first started day shift I got a patient and all I knew was that he was coming from a nursing home. He was an undocumented citizen. He was actually my age, was in a car accident and he was in a semi-vegetative state, quadriplegic from a spinal cord injury. He was being admitted from the nursing home. I took care of him every day. I was the new nurse so I got him for the total patient care experience. After like taking care of him and bathing him and talking to him he really started to come out of his shell over time. Working with him, we were eventually

able to get him up into a wheelchair and wheel him around and he started talking which was something he hadn't done and it was a good feeling knowing that my efforts really made a difference. It wasn't just me obviously. It was so cool. He stayed with us for 2 years though since he was undocumented. But it was just really cool to see what a difference you could make in somebody just through taking care of them. It was really cool. It validated why I'm a nurse and what I was doing was helpful because he was like an infant, he was crying and didn't talk and didn't look at anybody and it was wonderful for him that when his family visited him he could interact with them and they were all happy. So, it was just that he was one way and then he changed and transformed to being more of a person. It seemed like I made a difference, a positive difference in somebody. It changed me too cause I realized what I can do by my actions and not just my words, just by being present and building a trusting relationship, being there and telling him when I was coming and going, making sure I stopped in his room frequently and held his hand. In nursing school they tell you the rules, be clear, be present, be an active listener, do this, do this, do this and you hear it as an idea but you really don't have a chance to truly practice it in school. So, this was my first chance to actually see the cause and effect of what I did learn in

> school and what I do know as a person but on a different level. There something to be said for experiencing it on your own. He definitely taught me a lot too about myself and things like that. It was definitely a reciprocal relationship in the end. He just taught me the importance of being authentic and being, you know, obviously about the verbal communication and how important non-verbal is. He just taught me a lot about humor and he would sing "La cucaracha." It's a lot about how to keep humor and keep light of things and the importance of little things.

Beth had a difficult time describing a best day nursing. She asked a clarifying question, "an individual event?' She then described a nursing situation from the beginning of her nursing career 10 years ago. Beth declared, "It was just really cool to see what a difference you could make in somebody just through taking care of them. It was really cool." This beginning career nursing situation validated why she became a nurse and how she found joy in watching her patient progress. .

Beth had been working on a medical-surgical floor for 10 years and claimed it is the camaraderie with the other nurses that gets her through her day. She states "I really enjoy what I do; the patients keep me going. I really like what I do." She described how the patients keep her going as being energized by the patient.

Beth described that by doing sacred work she knew she was being helpful to her patient. She made a difference in her patient's life and it "validated why I am a nurse."

Beth creates the nursing situation when responding to the call and by being present as, "building a trusting relationship…making sure I stopped in his room frequently and held his hand." She was transformed by being present and intentionally being there with her patient. Beth described her nursing as humility and being open to grow and learn from the patient, anticipating what mattered most. "By taking the time to explain things, in a trusting relationship, they know my intentions and I feel validated."

Beth discovered that by bringing book learning of caring to her practice, she was able to apply what she learned, "I learned caring in school, but really didn't get a chance to practice it in school." Her patient taught her the importance of being authentic by being open to learn from her patient, "He taught me a lot about humor and keeping things light." She described how she learned from her patients, "it made me, I guess, a little more human in the fact that it was the reinforcement of the little things that you do and how important they are to people and that really did change me."

Beth claimed to be a big believer in taking breaks, if not she states "you are not going to be as effective I tell the nurses on the floor, you have to take a break. You have to care for self. You're not just there for yourself, you're there for other people, but I mean, people do not deserve you coming in with a bad attitude." By taking care of self in a reflective thoughtful practice, Beth takes the time to "sit down and get my thoughts together about what I really need to do."

Beth declared that what mattered most to her in her career right now is "just the same thing that mattered to me before, to really make a difference—to be there and to make a positive difference in somebody's life whether it's a small one or a big one or to help them along. So I hope when I become a nurse practitioner I can make a bigger difference because I will have a longer relationship with the patients."

Beth focused on coming to know the patient as a person, doing the best and being the best to make a difference, "I feel like I've done the best that I can be that day…my energy that I have put on to them." She described how she 'puts her energy' to the patient as an understanding of what makes them who they are. Beth stated that she works with them in a therapeutic relationship and begins by asking them what matters most.

Beth expressed how she appreciated being mentored, "some of the girls had charisma, they seemed to be getting things done and they would mentor me. They would say, 'OK, stop, just stop, now figure out what is going on with this patient', definitely prompting by the girls I worked with, it wasn't just all on me, it was the girls around me prompting and mentoring me to step back and reevaluate what I am doing."

Eleven categories emerged from the description of what is a best day at nursing practice for Beth and are presented with significant statements to support the category. A table is presented to facilitate clarity.

Table 8

Category Development—Participant #8: Beth

Significant Statement	Category
"…actually the beginning of my nursing career when I first started, I got a patient from a nursing home…he was my patient for two years."	Nursing as an Evolving Process
"Really cool to see what a difference you could make in somebody just through taking care of them…and having them come back to say hello."	Caring, finding joy in watching patient progress; Making a difference
"Validated why I'm a nurse and what I was doing was helpful."	Validation
"…by being present and building a trusting relationship…making sure I stopped in his room frequently and held his hand."	Creating the nursing situation with trust
"I learned caring in school, but really didn't get a chance to **<u>Table 8(*continues*)</u>**	Bringing book learning of *(table continues)*

practice it in school."	caring to practice
"He taught me the importance of being authentic and being…he taught me a lot about humor…and keep light of things and the importance of the little things."	Being open to learn from the patient through humility
"By taking the time to explain things in a trusting relationship, they know my intentions and I feel validated."	Trusting relationship
"The patients keep me going."	Being energized by the patient
"…let me make sure they are okay and let me sit down and get my thoughts together about what I really need to do."	Reflective, thoughtful practice
"I am a big believer in taking breaks…you got to get away from the phone, get something to eat, go to the bathroom."	Caring for self
"I feel like I've done the best that I can be that day…my energy that I have put on to them."	Focusing on coming to know the patient, doing the best, being the best
"…they seemed to be getting things done and they would mentor me."	Appreciating being mentored

Emerging Relational Themes

Relational Themes

The researcher identified four relational themes of being that emerged across the texts of this study: (1) Practicing from Inner Core Beliefs; (2) Understanding the Other from Within; (3) Making a Difference; and (4) Nursing as an Evolving Process. The four themes and the supporting categories are presented in Table 9.

Practicing from Inner Core Beliefs. The researcher interpreted Inner Core Beliefs from participants' descriptions of what keeps them in nursing. Inner core beliefs are defined as the basis of ethical caring focused on fulfilling the needs of others. Practicing from Inner Core Beliefs was interpreted as a reflective experience that reveals the beauty and complexity of caring for another as an unfolding of the day-to-dayness of nursing practice. The participants described being guided by ethical caring in complex nursing situations. By being in the right place, at the right time and doing the right thing, the participants described a loving spiritual experience. Doing the right thing is ethical caring and keeps the nurse in nursing by doing something of value, to give back and validates who the nurse is. It is meaningful for the nurse to make the world a better place one person at a time while valuing doing the right thing. Intentional nursing with a purpose gives the nurse a sense of worth by taking care of self in a reflective thoughtful practice that is spiritually guided. The nurse holds her or his own values by doing the right thing with an ethical stance.

Practicing from Inner Core Beliefs, as a Relational Theme, was interpreted from categories including caring as the ethical thing to do, spiritually guiding self and other, respect for other, valuing as personal beliefs, reflective experience and intentionality.

Understanding the Other from Within. The researcher interpreted this relational theme as the mutuality of finding grace in the other as the beginning point of coming to know and understand the other in the caring relationship. The nurse shares compassion within the nursing situation by creating the caring encounter in the best situation possible. The participants appreciated hope and found joy in their nursing practice by encouraging hope in the one nursed. The participants described experiencing compassion by "walking in their patient's shoes" which seemed to make extraordinary things happen. Nurses respond to the calls for nursing uniquely and also send out calls of compassionate presence. Understanding the accepted culture of caring for other and caring for self, the participants come to know self as nurse who is able to make a difference with compassionate presence. Within the nursing situation the nursed and nurse share the celebration of their mutual reciprocal relationship of nurturance and caring.

Understanding the Other from Within grew from categories including reciprocal relationships, appreciating, finding joy, celebration, hoping, coming to know, called to, sending out the call, respond to call and compassion.

Making a Difference. Each participant revealed the importance of making a difference in someone's life. The participants declared that making a difference was an energizing passion described as joy, a personal high and satisfaction. The nurses experienced that making a difference is validating as "what I do" and "who I am." What each nurse brings to the patient's life is who she or he, the nurse, is. By making a difference, each nurse validates who she or he is, what she or he does, and this experience is grounding. One participant stated "it's integral to who I am, it's feeling that I am doing something of value, giving back, and its part of making the world a better place one person at a time while healing the world." Another declared, "I may not make a difference in everybody's life, but at least once a day I make a difference in somebody's life." The experience of making a difference is a feeling of being energized. The nurse participants felt energized by caring, exhibited by a sense of satisfaction as they help someone through intentional knowing.

Making a Difference as a Relational Theme was interpreted from categories including doing, caring for, mentoring, competence, confidence, sense of satisfaction, validation and energizing.

Nursing as an Evolving Process. The participants offered that they have experienced many best days in practice, so much so that they found it difficult to describe only one nursing situation. Each participant needed a long silent reflective pause to gather thoughts about one nursing situation that could represent a best day in practice. All participants described that there were so many important nursing situations over time of their nursing career. Some participants returned to when they were first nursing over 10 years ago, and a few over 28 years ago. One participant described a nursing situation that occurred over a two year period.

The researcher interpreted Nursing as an Evolving Process of creating the nursing situations with openness and willingness to enter the world of the other to understand the wholeness of the person. The participants described the knowledge they possess and the trust they are given from the patient as a process. The nurse participants respond to the call with intentional knowing of the other as patient and person as whole, providing an ongoing presence as an environment of healing. Humility is the grounding for intentional knowing.

Nursing as an evolving process as a relational theme, was interpreted from categories including nursing situation over time, openness, wholeness, courage, trust, humility, caring response and willingness.

The following Table is provided to illustrate the relational themes and supporting categories.

Table 9

Relational Themes and Supporting Categories

Relational Themes	Supporting Categories
Practicing from inner core beliefs	Ethical caring Spiritual guiding Respect for the other Valuing Reflective experience Intentionality
Understanding the other from within relationships	Appreciating Finding joy, celebration Hoping Coming to know Called to Sending out the call Respond to the call Compassion
Making a difference	Doing Caring for Mentoring Competence Confidence Sense of satisfaction Validation Energizing
Nursing as an evolving process over time	Nursing situations Openness *(table continues)*

Table 9 (*continues*)	Wholeness Courage Trust Humility Caring response Willingness

The overall meaning of what keeps nurses in nursing for the eight participants in this study was interpreted from the four Relational Themes: Practicing from Inner Core Beliefs, Understanding the Other from Within, Making a Difference and Nursing as an Evolving Process. The overall meaning is described as a constitutive pattern which the researcher has named *Intentional Compassion Energy*.

The participants in this study reflected on and described the meaning of what keeps nurses in nursing and their accounts brought the concept of compassion energy to life. Dunn (2007) conceptualized compassion energy through the lens of caring theory and used a caring concept clarification process. The conceptual synthesis of compassion energy identified three attributes: compassionate presence, patterned nurturance and intentionally knowing the nursed and self as whole.

The nurses in this study describe initiating the experience of compassion energy when they answer the call from a patient. When the nurse answers the call of the nursed with the intent to alleviate suffering or celebrating joy, the nursed reveals her or his hopes, dreams and aspirations. The nurse's and nursed's individual expressions of affirmation, support and celebration are exchanged as energy via compassionate presence. Compassion becomes the energy of caring.

In the nursing situation, the nurse answers the call with pattered nurturance which yields energy to be compassionately present. The dynamic unfolding of the energy exchange is experienced as patterned nurturance through listening, knowing and being with the nursed in authentic compassionate presence (Swanson, 1991; Watson, 2006). In the context of the nursing situation, there is a vibrational centering which is meaningful and nourishes nurturance. This energy patterning is depicted as patterned nurturance (Todaro-Franceschi, 1999).

In intentional caring consciousness, the nurse intentionally knows the nursed as whole. The patient has the choice of letting the nurse know her or him as person (Boykin & Schoenhofer, 2001; Locsin, 1998). Compassion energy is the intersubjective gift of compassion that gives nurses the opportunity to be with the nursed. Alleviating suffering or celebrating joy, the nurse and the nursed express a warm approval while sharing joyful satisfaction in the nursing situation by enhancing compassionate presence, patterned nurturance and intentionally knowing the nursed and self as whole (Dunn, 2007). Thus, intentional compassion energy is defined as the regeneration of nurses' capacity to foster interconnectedness when the nurse activates the intent to nurse (Dunn, 2009).

This study revealed that intention grounded the nurse participants' practice as intentional compassion energy. Each participant revealed that it was through conscious intention to create the nursing situation with the intent to be compassionately present that allowed them to come to know the patient through patterned nurturance.

Evaluation Criteria

Evaluation criteria were provided by Lincoln and Guba (1985) and elaborated by Sandelowski (1986) for examination of the findings in this study. Lincoln and Guba (1985) describe rigor as trustworthiness and authenticity. Trustworthiness enabled interpretative inquiry to make a reasonable claim to this study's methodological soundness and has established rigor by using techniques that provide truth-value through credibility, applicability through transferability, consistency through dependability and neutrality through confirmability (Sandelowski, 1986). Authenticity described the mechanism by which I ensured that the findings of the study are real, true and authentic (Lincoln & Guba, 1985).

Truth-Value Through Credibility

I remained opened to discovery in listening to the voices and words from the participants. Heideggarian hermeuneutics methodology is the interpretive research instrument that measures the phenomenon as it is defined in this study. The core principle of hermeneutics is that understanding is a process that is achieved by comparison. I compared parts of the text with the whole. The meaning of the text was compared with the historical or situatedness of the participant. The text was then compared with my own background and then again with the method expert from the dissertation committee. Understanding and meaning therefore had a circular nature. *Applicability Through Transferability*

A convenience sample of eight registered nurses were recruited, all were unknown to the researcher. The findings were meaningful and the results were checked with two randomly selected participants. The selected participant's experiences will be shared so that the participant readers of the research findings can evaluate their own experiences.

Consistency Through Dependability

The dissertation chair and research committee members can follow the audit trail in regards to theme analysis from the transcribed interviews.

Neutrality Through Confirmability

I was engaged with the participants, however neutral in reporting of the research findings. I described the findings from the participant's voice and viewpoint, while motivated to learn new perspectives from nurses regarding what keeps them nursing and to share this knowledge with others.

Intentional Compassion Energy is the interpretive finding of "What Keeps Nurses in Nursing" for the eight participants in this study which illuminates the meaning of Being in the everydayness of nursing practice. Each of the eight participants expressed experiences of ethical caring values from inner core beliefs. Compassionate caring attributes were provided as understanding the other from within, as an example one participant stated "I walked in her shoes." The lived experience of what it means to make a difference to each participant was discussed. Lastly, nursing as an evolving process was experienced as day-to-dayness of creating nursing situations over time.

Heidegger (1927/1962) offers three elements of Being as a guide to understanding the complexity of Being. Each person is within the context of her everyday practices, concerns, and things that matter. The researcher compared a part of the text with the whole. The meaning of the text was then compared with the historical or situatedness of the participant. The text was also compared with the researcher's own background. The intent of the researcher was to elucidate the nature of being human in the experience that held personal meaning while nursing another. The process doing this method is written as it was experienced by this researcher while immersed in the hermeneutic circle and it is described as it was lived.

> I listen to the voices of my participants face to face during the interviews as an honored person seated in the concert hall "front row center." I listen and re-listen to their sage experiences and immediately identify with their joy of nursing. The sound of each syllable, word, slang, nurse-speak, phrase, sentence and paragraph is music to my ears. I listen intently while transcribing each 'ummm' and 'you know' while appreciating their long deep quiet reflective thoughtful pauses. The text from their voices lay before me. I took their voices everywhere, in the car driving, walking my dog, reading Heideggerian philosophy inspired to think, write and find meaning, to make visible the invisible. I listen for the meaning in other literary sources and cultural expressions for a deeper understanding. I have been re-listening, re-reading, re-writing, re-thinking, re-saying and reflecting on their words and my interpretation of them. It becomes both simple and difficult at the same time as I spiral into revision after revision. I take comfort in re-experiencing the past with an orientation towards the future while interpreting

> their meaning in the moment. I think of myself as a sage nurse too, that the meaning of Being nurse is always already available and is itself a positive phenomenon which needs elucidation. I come to appreciate the wisdom of my participants as they are the expert voice to tell the story of what keeps them in nursing.

This ontological interpretative perspective explores the nurse-self as what it means to be. The authentic self chooses to live with actions arising from self rather than conforming to routine for the sake of routine. Person moves in authentic time from past to future in the course of the present moment, considers self, chooses with wholeness of being, and in doing so, achieves an authentic way of life (Heidegger, 1927/1962). The findings of this study reveal the authentic way of life for the nurse participants described as a constitutive pattern named *Intentional Compassion Energy.*

Chapter Summary

The findings presented in the chapter are the results of a Heideggerian hermeneutical phenomenology inquiry into the experience of what keeps nurses in nursing for eight practicing registered nurses. This study unfolded in a nursing program at a state university in southeastern United States.

This purposive sample consisted of eight participants who were students at a state university in southeastern United States. A flyer was distributed to the faulty and brief presentations were conducted at the beginning of class. Eight students emailed the researcher with their interest and intent to participate voluntarily in this study. The participants contacted the researcher by email and included their phone number to schedule an appointment to be interviewed. The participants were unknown to the researcher and volunteered to be interviewed. However, as described earlier, the subjects were all students of varying levels in an educational program at the time of their participation in the study. Therefore, it is possible that they were more finely tuned to philosophic considerations than might be the case with participants not currently enrolled in school.

Data were collected during one semi-structured interview lasting approximately one hour. Target questions included: Tell me a nursing situation about your best day in practice. What keeps you in nursing? Why would you want to stay in nursing, what would make you leave? What matters most to you at this time? Other probing questions were asked during the interviews to elicit a fuller description.

The interviews were audio taped and transcribed verbatim. Confidentiality has been maintained using pseudonyms for the participants. Diekelmann and Allen (1989) provided the seven stage process for data analysis. Stage 1: Reading the transcripts from the audio taped interviews in order to obtain an overall understanding of the text by looking for the dialectic within the text itself; Stage 2: Each text was summarized and significant statements were extracted as descriptive statements. Each interpretative exemplar was intended to illuminate the meaning of what keeps nurses in nursing from the participant's perspective. The statements were in the participant's words. Initially 71 significant statements were provided to explore the meaning of language and Being; Stage 3: The descriptive statements were interpreted into 31 categories. The researcher was opened and engaged into the hermeneutic circle of understanding and interpreting by re-listening, re-reading, re-thinking, re-saying, and re-writing. The categories developed and the researcher identified composite analytic themes that recurred and reflected shared practice and common meanings; Stage 4: The texts were re-read and examined for meaning and relationships to clarify and identify relational themes. The themes represent the relationship of the categories across the texts. The four relational themes that emerged from the categories are: Practicing from inner core beliefs; Understanding the other from within; Making a difference; and Nursing as an evolving process. Stage 5: As themes are compared, a constitutive pattern that links the themes emerged. The interpreted findings of this study emerged from the descriptive statements, developed categories, analyzed and synthesized themes. The overall meaning is described as a constitutive pattern named *Intentional Compassion Energy*. Stage 6: The data analysis is validated with the dissertation committee member who is familiar with both the content and the research method. These findings illuminated the participants discovering the meaning of Being in the everydayness of nursing practice; and Stage 7: A full description of the experience of what keeps nurses in nursing has been developed and completed.

Evaluation criteria was provided by Lincoln and Guba (1985) and elaborated by Sandowloski (1986) has been utilized for the examination of the findings in this study. The criteria include: credibility, transferability, dependability, and confirmability.

This summary provided a review of the study, the participants, data analysis and evaluation criteria.

CHAPTER 5

DISCUSSION AND IMPLICATIONS

> … I cared for him and I made a difference in his life. I cared for his soul, body, person, dreams, ideas, and after all was done, he thanked me for being present. I went home that night feeling overwhelmed with the love I have for my profession, and how Mr. O helped me more than I helped him. (Roccio G. Vinas, personal communication, July 1, 2008)

This chapter presents a summary of the findings of this study and the interpretation of those findings. Implications of the findings for nursing practice, education, health policy and recommendations for future nursing research are offered. Recommendations for additional studies on this topic are suggested.

This research study was conducted to discover what keeps nurses in nursing? Eight participants in this study described nursing situations that revealed how they experienced a best day nursing. The researcher interpreted the findings in this study to illuminate the constitutive meaning of what keeps nurses in nursing and has named that phenomenon *Intentional Compassion Energy*.

The researcher described the methodological and theoretical framework as a model for implications for nursing practice. The overall implications for nursing practice are discussed under the following headings: Practicing From Inner Core Beliefs, Understanding the Other From Within, Making A Difference and Nursing as an Evolving Process. The results of this study are discussed in terms of practice, education, policy and future research.

The nursing shortage is impacted by the aging workforce, increased professional opportunities for women, decreased enrollment in nursing programs, shortage of nursing faculty and the aging population (AACN, 2008). Several factors are associated with the workplace environment that results in job dissatisfaction. They include things such as violence in the workplace, understaffing and an increase in non-nursing duties (Evans, 2005; Jackson et al., 2002; O'Brien-Pallas et al., 2004). Most of this research, however, has been investigated from a quantitative perspective and takes a negative focus, that is, what is wrong with nursing. Little is qualitatively known about the positive view: what keeps nurses in nursing. Studying what keeps nurses in nursing from Boykin and Schoenhofers (2001) Nursing As Caring theoretical framework and Heideggerian hermeneutic methodological inquiry provided insight into approaches useful for promoting retention of a quality caring and compassionate nursing workforce.

Studies convey that nurses do not have the time to provide the compassionate care they desire to realize (Abenroth & Flannery, 2006; Cowin & Henstberger-Sims, 2005; Sabo, 2006). Nursing is more demanding and multifaceted than it has ever been. The demand on nurses continues to increase due to patient acuity, changes in reimbursement, access to care and technology (Christmas, 2008).

Each participant in this study expressed feelings of making a difference with compassionate caring as an unfolding process which is experienced as day-to-dayness while practicing from inner core beliefs. The essence of this phenomenon is ontological and answers the question of what keeps nurses in nursing. The participants' historical context and world view situates them in the moment of space and time to experience clearly who they are through their lived experience. This understanding of who the participants are is seen and understood in everyday experiences. Nurses are ordinary people situated in extraordinary circumstances.

The researcher interpreted the nurses' experience to discover the meaning of being in the everydayness. The expression of caring work using the nurse's voice for interpretation of the nature of her or his truth, language, thinking, dwelling and being brings the profession to a better understanding of what it takes to continue to nurse in light of the looming nursing shortage.

The researcher identified the following relational themes analyzed from this study: Practicing from Inner Core Beliefs, Understanding the Other from Within, Making a Difference and Nursing as an Evolving Process. The researcher identified the interpretive meaning that emerged from the synthesis of the relational themes as the lived experience of what keeps nurses in nursing, that the researcher named intentional compassion energy. These findings contribute to new knowledge which may influence a sea change from a social contract relationship towards a covenantal relationship between nurse and the one nursed. This new relationship will include a willingness to enter openly, wherein the concealed will be revealed.

Implications for Nursing Practice

The nursing situation is an interactive qualitative place to dwell and study the dynamic and evolving energetic process of compassion. For the nurse, in the context of the nursing situation, meaning and purpose was explored through a Heideggerian hermeneutic interpretive phenomenological method of what is it that keeps the nurse nursing at the bedside, curbside, under trees or wherever nursing takes place. The participants described how they intentionally made themselves available to their patients. Nurses send out the call to persons by being available and making the nurse-patient relationship a nurturing and caring place (Lesniak, 2008). The nurse participants in this study explained that they appreciate the present moment and they cultivate an intimate relationship with patients by being purposeful (Intentional) in making a difference, giving them a sense of satisfaction in their nursing practice.

Practicing From Inner Core Beliefs

Intentional compassion energy occurs when the nurse values the uniqueness of answering the call with compassionate presence, patterned nurturance, and intentionally knowing the patient and self as whole (Dunn, 2007). Each of the participants expressed that her or his nursing practice emerges from an inner core belief which is considered an ethical caring value. Woods' (1999) grounded theory examination of the everyday moral decision making of experienced nurses suggested that maintenance of a nursing ethic is a core variable. Every moral decision inspires an action essential in everyday nursing practice. Exposure to good nursing practice in the form of ethical role models and mentoring may guide the novice nurse in a process over time to develop an understanding of the essential ethical requirements of nursing practice. Most of the participants in this study described nursing practice as a spiritual understanding of the human person as created in the image of God. Further, they viewed the body as a living unity and expressed that the Holy Spirit guides the nurse's work. The spiritual perspective identified in nursing practice is the connectedness with others, the universe or God, a belief in something greater than self and the creative energy that unfolds as a dynamic process (Allen-Shelly & Miller, 2006).

Understanding the Other From Within

Caring theory informs nurses to nurture professional values. Upholding caring values in nurses' practice helps the nurse to transcend from a state where nursing is perceived as 'just a job' to a state in which nursing is considered a profession of great humanistic importance. With such a mind set, the nurse will learn that to provide compassion to ease patients' and families' suffering, and to promote health, will contribute to expansion of the nurse's own actualization. This leads to a conscious caring attempt to make an intentional conscious effort to care for self, and the patient and family, compassionately. Schantz (2007) clarified the meaning of the concept of compassion and examined its relevance in the context of everyday practice. She asserted that is it necessary to identify, understand and internalize the meaning of compassion. Then, the next step is to exercise compassion in nursing practice every day (Schantz, 2007, p. 54).

Nurses enter into a partnership with the one nursed and engage in meaningful dialogue as the dynamic pattern unfolds (Newman, 1994, 2008). What matters most to the patient becomes transparent as the patient guides the discussion. The nurse projects back to the patient what is heard with a mutual vibrational resonance (Newman, 1994; Rogers, 1970). The patient determines what is important through an energy exchange with the authentic presence of a caring other, the compassionate nurse (Boykin & Schoenhofer, 2001; Newman, 1994; Rogers, 1970).

Making a Difference

The participants in this study described the experience of being able to make a difference in a person's life while feeling a sense of satisfaction that energized their nursing practice. When the nurse intends to be caring she or he initiates an energy exchange that promotes compassion energy and prevents experiencing compassion fatigue or burnout (Dunn, 2009). Human beings live in the world with meaningful compassionate relationships. This researcher believes that the culture of nursing should be considered and nurtured as compassion in present day practice. Compassion culture in the nursing environment could focus on being culturally accepted by discovering the meaning of making a difference in patients' everydayness. Nurses will grow and thrive if they understand how to self-generate vigor as intentional compassion energy (Dunn, 2009).

Simms et al. (1990) explored work excitement in nursing to describe nurses who do well and enjoy their work. Work excitement was defined by Simms and associates (1990) as, "personal enthusiasm and commitment for work, evidenced by creativity, receptivity to learning and ability to see opportunity in everyday situations" (p. 178). The participants in this study described how making a difference in a patient's life energizes the nurse participant and gives meaning to their nursing. Just as the meaning is revealed in being, the essence of nursing is revealed in the being and doing of nursing. Exploring intentional compassion energy through research will contribute to the body of nursing knowledge and practice that can make a difference in a person's life, the nurse's life and the nursing profession as a whole.

Nursing as an Evolving Process

The purpose of this study was to explore what keeps nurses in nursing, by examining relational experiences between the nurse and patient in the context of the nursing situation. Each participant had difficulty describing only one nursing situation about a good day in nursing as they looked at their entire nursing experience and career to describe a good day in practice over time. The participants in this study described their love for nursing as a process that keeps them in nursing.

The evolving process constitutes places and spaces for experience, reflecting the complexity of each patient-nurse relationship. Nursing as an evolving process is simplistic, yet complex, and involves a continuous search for self-knowledge, fulfillment, pleasure and courage of health and well-being. At the same time there are situations full of sadness and illness that relate to the loss of possibilities, leaving both the patient and the nurse vulnerable. The patient's illness can interrupt plans and modify roles without previous preparation. By discovering openness and willingness as creative resources, nurses find nursing as an evolving process to be inspiring.

In the past two decades, scholars have been redefining nursing in the nurse-patient-family-environment relationship, emphasizing intimacy as its vehicle for effective delivery of care. The prevalence of biomedical structures, disease labeling and technological tasks has fostered an environment which has made it possible for health care providers to practice detachment under the banner of professionalism (Sanghavi, 2006). The participants in this study described an intentional initiation of action to alleviate suffering with a willingness to go beyond what was expected, giving the gift of self, time, or actions for the person in need. In giving this gift, the participants received a gift in return as satisfaction and gratification experienced by a personal high, passion, celebration, and energy.

Educational Implications

The participants in this study reported feelings of compassion resulting from identification and acknowledgement of suffering. Along with the acknowledgement of suffering comes the urge to act on it, share it and abate it (Schantz, 2007). Given the opportunity to rise to the occasion and use compassion as strength, nurses can have courage and learn how to become more politically active in conflict resolution. Nurses can work to prevent natural and man made disasters at the local, community, national and international levels.

Overcoming the tendency to care at a distance requires a new discourse. Nurses should investigate Heidegger's idea of empty busywork in which the nurse may use technology as a barrier against developing a relationship with the patient (Heidegger, 1927/1962; Locsin, 1998). Nurses can assist the patient in the work of suffering by understanding how to be compassionately present.

Being present with another who is suffering is an important part of the healing process for those who seek meaning in their life. Teaching nursing students to focus their intent on compassionate caring to trigger the energy exchange, rather than focusing on task oriented "doing the job" or "getting tasks done" should be implemented into academic curricula and orientation programs in the workplace. Swenson and Sims (2007) argue that nursing is interpretive in nature as nurses' focus on the ones nursed and their unique experiences. Swenson and Sims (2007) state that,

> Narrative-Centered Curriculum focuses on seeking, hearing, responding to, reflecting on, and interpreting clinical and personal stories of students, patients, preceptors and teachers. The Narrative-Centered

> Curriculum enables teachers to 'put their minds where their hearts are' in the realm of teaching and learning and to use pedagogical approaches for both a scientific and phenomenological and experiential view of the world of clinical practice. (p. 156)

Narratives enable the one nursed to share an experience with the nurse who did not have access to the experience. Presently, education is focused on care, cure, and restorative function and does not address 'relief of suffering' adequately (Swenson & Sims, 2007). Narrative education is considered the phenomenology of human suffering which assists students in learning to dwell patiently, humbly and attentively with the suffering nursed (Swenson & Sims, 2007). Integrating substantive philosophical content in nursing education curricula will enable students to come to know what it means to be human and to suffer. Students will thereby have an opportunity for deep reflection, intense dialogue and meaningful research.

Critical reflection using narrative story is a way of gaining self-awareness and personal growth, as well as the notion that caring can be learned through reflection. There is a philosophical link between self-care, caring and holistic nursing practice (Wilson & Grams, 2007). The process of self-reflection is a way to gain self-awareness and learn to care for self. Sherwood (1997b) acknowledged the importance of a caring connection centered on caring for self.

The participants in this study expressed the importance of allowing nurses time to care-for-self. Compassionate self-care enhanced their sense of passion, meaning and purpose at work. Nursing has put forth efforts toward recognizing the complexity and significance of the concepts of care and caring, Compassionate care is not simply taking the pain or suffering away from the other. It entails entering into the other's experience so as to share the burden with them in order to help them retain their dignity. Nurses will nurture their own intrinsic ethical and spiritual values by caring for self and be available to send out the call for a nurturing and caring relationship.

As an example, "Caring for Self" is a 15-week elective course offered to students across campus and taught by nursing faculty at a southeastern public university. The course focuses on experiential learning and requires active participation by all students. Topics include a wide variety of complementary modalities to enhance physical, spiritual, and emotional health and well-being, such as aromatherapy, meditation and yoga. A variety of creative exercises enhance the participant's personal sense of creativity and self-esteem, such as, role playing, drawing and treasure maps. Journaling is another requirement for this course. The student's prior life journey may not have been health promoting and may have detracted from enhancing one's own sense of self (St. Pierre, 2006). St. Pierre (2006) discovered, through a content analysis in a descriptive qualitative study, that nursing students indicated a profound change in beliefs about caring for self after the course. Their attitudes shifted regarding the importance of caring for self, as well as giving permission to one's self to participate in self-care activities.

Recommendations for Future Nursing Research

New questions about what keeps nurses in nursing evolved from the findings of this study. The themes that emerged from the participants' voices provided a conceptualization of intentional compassion energy as practicing from inner core beliefs, understanding the other from within, while making a difference as nursing care evolves as an ethical, spiritual, compassionate, energizing caring process. Future nursing research in relation to the findings is suggested here.

The study uncovered the need for additional research in several areas including the rewards of nursing, the use and effectiveness of compassionate caring mentoring, and caring nurse ethics. More importantly, asking nurses what they value in their profession and how their work lives can enable them to act on their values would generate useful knowledge in developing recruitment and retention strategies to attract and retain qualified caring and compassionate nurses.

Quantitative and qualitative research methods to study intentional compassion energy will add to the body of nursing knowledge. Quantitative research methods will describe how prevalent, how often and what are the characteristics of intentional compassion energy. Identifying factors that relate to compassion energy and naming their antecedents can be analyzed (Creswell, 2003). Measurable associations among factors can be explained in a quantitative study that can predict what will happen if intentional compassion energy is altered or enhanced or if an intervention is introduced, such as a particular educational endeavor (Dunn, 2009)..

Benner (1984) described clinical knowledge as an interpretative approach. The intentions and understanding of the participants are taken into consideration and seen as dependent on a shared world of meaning (Benner, 1984, p. 40). The novice nurse's interpretation of compassion compared to the expert nurse's could be examined with ethnographical field work methods. Researchers can learn from members of the nursing culture regarding differences and similarities when providing compassionate care. The assumption is that all nurses desire to care with compassion (Dunn, 2009). Even if the impulse of compassion attracts people to nursing, it is not always translated into action. In the past, improving quality care meant focusing on racial and geographic disparities, patient safety and adherence to clinical guidelines, but not compassion. Most interventions to improve compassion primarily target students. What is missing is a method of research to continually reinforce the positive aspects of compassion among practicing registered nurses (Salvage, 2006; Sanghavi, 2006).

Nursing situations present the novice nurse with a set of tasks that must be accomplished (Benner et al., 1996). Overwhelmed by the biomedical needs of the patient, novice nurses may feel unable to attend to the psychosocial needs. A qualitative field study of novice nurses who successfully provide technical care, such as measuring and documenting fluid output from patients having multiple drainage tubes, will provide an opportunity for them to discuss their experience.

The novice nurses will make a conscious effort to offer their presence and compassion during the next scheduled time to measure and document the patient drainage tube output. Thus they will intentionally focus on the patient while obtaining the outputs, and then discuss their experiences, comparing the task-focused encounter to the patient-focused encounter. Such information will yield data for intentional compassion energy theory building and for nursing practice (Dunn, 2009). The nursing situation is an interactive qualitative place to dwell and study the dynamic and evolving energetic process of compassion.

Policy

Major health care reform discussion is occurring on the national scene as this dissertation is being completed. This researcher hopes that the discussion will include efforts to ensure that health care systems consider the humanness of those they serve. Nurses explore the case for development of qualities of creativity, compassion, self-realization and judgment in nursing practice. Unfortunately most health care reform discussions focus on finances, number of people covered, sources of payment, and other non-human concerns. Nursing leaders in the Institute of Medicine, such as Linda Aiken, document social, economic, and environmental factors that impinge on nursing practice (Aiken, et al., 2001, 2002). In effect, nurse health policy researchers argue the importance of nurses to provide humanistic understanding and discovery for effective health care. The dilemma is between the structure of health care and the structure of human social life.

In order to connect to the human condition, knowledge of what it means to be human is required. Part of that knowledge lies in awakening nurses' ethical consciousness and compassion that unfolds as caring for self and caring for others. The ethical component of nursing is focused on matters of what ought to be done (Carper, 1978). Voluntary actions are guided by a judgment of the right thing to do personally and professionally. Nurses should be active participants in the development of policies from individual bedsides to hospital-wide to system encompassing methods designed to promote patient safety, reduce medical errors and address environmental system factors and human factors that present risk to patients (ANA, 2003, p. 11). Specific departments or units could support professional nurses and the work environment that reflects an attitude of values attached to positive nursing action that facilitates choice.

Developing a deliberate plan of action on the unit level will guide decisions and achieve rational processes for nurses to be enabled to "do the right thing." Policy merely guides actions toward those that are most likely to achieve a desired outcome. A research study could be developed to describe key social, psychological and structural processes that occur in the nursing situation in a health care setting. It could focus on a developing social experience of an important health care event or episode. Discovery of a core belief that is central to explain what is going on is grounded in reality for the nurse and nursed and could be identified. The aim is to understand perspectives, perceptions, meaning, and uniqueness of the subjective lives of the nurse and nursed and what is occurring between them in the encounter of the nursing situation. The study will explain the nursing responses to the suffering nursed within the context of the nursing situation. This study could suggest adding moral voice of a nursing ethic to promote good nursing (Woods, 1999). Nurses value answering the call to nurse with compassionate presence, patterned nurturance and intentionally knowing the nursed and self as whole (Dunn 2007).

Thoughtful reflection of the nursing situation is interpretative and views the social phenomenon holistically. The patient and nurse together decide on their relationship as the patient determines the unique meaning which the experience of health, illness, suffering or dying is for that individual. Advocacy is based on the principle of freedom of self-determination. Patients are assisted by nurses to authentically exercise their freedom of self-determinism and choice based on their own values (Gadow, 1990). By assuring that a policy is in place to understand and promote the culture of compassion as the energy of caring nurses, peers and administrators will be aware and nurture this in the work environment.

Summary

This qualitative research study examined what keeps nurses in nursing. The eight registered nurses who participated in this study provided rich descriptive data from which four relational themes emerged: Practicing from Inner Core Beliefs, Understanding the Other from Within, Making a Difference and Nursing as an Evolving Process. The hermeneutical interpretative process guided the researcher to synthesize the themes into a constitutive pattern of meaning named *Intentional Compassion Energy.*

Intentional compassion energy was discovered in the meaning of the nurse participants' being in their everydayness of practice. The participants in this study described the intention to care compassionately as the grounding of their practice, striving to understand the other, to make a difference while living their nursing as an evolving process. Hermeneutic phenomenology provided the opening to discover what keeps nurses in nursing.

APPENDIX

A. Demographics

Participant	Age	Ethnicity	Years in Nursing	Specialty Area	Highest Earned Degree	Current Program of Study
109	54	Caucasian	33	L&D	BSN	MSN-ADM
209	49	Caucasian	29	NICU	BSN	MSN
309	49	Caucasian	28	Oncology	BSN	MSN-ED
409	28	Caucasian	5.5	Discharge	BSN	MSN
509	52	Caucasian	31	Community	MPH, RN	PhD
609	22	Afro-Carribean	1.5	Ortho-Surg	AD	BSN
709	27	Afro-American	6	Education	BSN	MSN-ED
809	31	Caucasian	10	Med-Surg	BSN	MSN-FNP

B. Interview Guide

Tell me a nursing situation about your best day in practice.

What keeps you in nursing?

Why would you want to stay in nursing, what would make you leave?

What matters most to you at this time?

What are your hopes and dreams for the future?

Tell me how you experience nursing.

Does the relationship between the nurse and patient have an impact on registered nurses intent to stay?

Bibliography

Abendroth, M., & Flannery, J. (2006). Predicting the risk of compassion fatigue: A study of hospice nurses. *Journal of Hospice and Palliative Nursing, 8*(6), 346-356.

Adams, R. E., Figley, C. R., & Boscarino, J. A. (2008). The compassion fatigue scale: Its use with social workers following urban disaster. *Research on Social Work Practice, 18*(3), 238-250.

Aiken, L. H., Clarke, S. P., Sloane, & Sochalski, J. (2001). Nurses' report on hospital quality of care and working conditions in five countries. *Health Affairs, 20*(3), 43-53.

Aiken, L. H., Clarke, S. P., Sloane, S. P., Sochalski, J., & Silber, J. H. (2002). Hospital nurse staffing and mortality, nurse burnout and job dissatisfaction. *JAMA* 288, 1987-1993.

Allen-Shelly, J., & Miller, A. B. (2006). *Called to care: A Christian worldview for nursing.* Downers Grove, IL: InterVarsity Press.

American Association of Colleges of Nursing. (2008). *Nursing Shortage Fact Sheet.* Retrieved January 26, 2009 from http://www.aacn.nche.edu/Media/FactSheets/NursingShortage.htm

Error! Hyperlink reference not valid.*American Heritage Dictionary of the English Language (*4th ed.*)*. Retrieved June 9, 2008, from http://dictionary.reference.com/browse/intentionality

American Nurses Association. (2001). Nurses concerned over working conditions, decline in quality of care. *ANA Survey, 14*(1), 1.

Baer, E. D. (1992). American nursing: 100 years of conflicting ideas and ideals. *Journal of the New York State Nurses Association, 23*(3), 16-21.

Beaudoin, L. E., & Edgar, L. (2003). Hassles: Their importance to nurses' quality of work life. *Nursing Economics, 21*(3), 106-113.

Benner, P. (1984). *From novice to expert: Excellence and power in clinical nursing practice.* Menlo Park, CA: Addison-Wesley.

Benner, P., Tanner, C. A., & Chesla, C. A. (1996). *Expertise in nursing practice: Caring, clinical judgment and ethics.* New York: Springer.

Benner, P. & Wrubel, J. (1989). *The primacy of caring: Stress and coping in health and illness*. Menlo Park, CA: Addison-Wesley.

Boykin, A., & Schoenhofer, S. (2001). *Nursing as caring: A model for transforming practice.* Sudbury, CT: NLN.

Boykin, A., & Schoenhofer, S. O. (2006). Anne Boykin and Savina O. Schoenhofer's Nursing as Caring Theory. In M. E. Parker (Ed.), *Nursing theories & nursing practice* (2nd ed.; pp. 334-348). Philadelphia: F. A. Davis.

Brilowski, G. A., & Wendler, M. C. (2004). An evolutionary concept analysis of caring. *Journal of Advanced Nursing, 50*(6), 641-650.

Buerhaus, P. I. (2007). Trends in the experiences of hospital-employed registered nurses: Results from three national surveys. *Nursing Economics, 25*(2), 69-80.

Buerhaus, P. I. (2008) Current and future state of the US nursing workforce. *JAMA, 300*(20), 2422-2424.

Buerhaus, P. I., Donelan, K., Ulrich, B. T., Norman, L., & Dittus, R. (2006). State of the registered nurse workforce in the U.S.. *Nursing Economics, 24*(1), 6-12.

Byrne, D., & McMurray, A. (1997). Caring for the dying: Nurses' experiences in hospice care. *Australian Journal of Advanced Nursing, 15*, 4-11.

Carper, B. A. (1978). Fundamental patterns of knowing in nursing. *Advances in Nursing Science, 1*(1), 13-20.

Christmas, K. (2008). How work environment impacts retention. *Nursing Economics*, *26*(5) 316-318.

Clark, M., & Giorgio, S. (1998). Nurses, indirect trauma and prevention. *Journal of Nursing Scholarship, 30,* 85-87.

Cohen, M. Z., Kahn, D. L., & Steeves, R. H. (2000). *Hermeneutic phenomenological research: A practical guide for nurse researchers.* Thousand Oaks, CA: Sage.

Collins, S., & Long, A. (2003). Too tired to care? The psychological effects of working with trauma. *Journal of Psychiatric Mental Health Nursing, 10,* 17-27.

Cowin, L. S., & Hengstberger-Sims, C. (2005). New graduate nurse self-concept and retention: A longitudinal survey. *International Journal of Nursing Studies, 43*(1), 59-70.

Creswell, J. W. (2003). *Research design: Qualitative, Quantitative and mixed methods approach* (2nd ed.). Thousand Oaks, CA: Sage.

Diekelmann, N. L., & Allen, D. G. (1989). A hermeneutic analysis of the NLN criteria for the appraisal of baccalaureate programs. In N. Diekelmann, D. Allen, & C. Tanner, *The NLN criteria for appraisal of baccalaurareate programs: A critical hermeneutic analysis* (pp. 11-13.). New York: NLN.

Dilthey, W. (1976). *Selected writings* (H. P. Rickman, Trans.). Cambridge, Great Britain: Cambridge University Press.

Draucker, C. B. (1999). The critique of Heideggerian hermeneutical nursing research. *Journal of Advanced Nursing, 30*(2), 360-373.

Dreyfus, H. L. (1994). *Being-in-the-world.* Cambridge, MA: MIT Press.

Dunn, D. J. (2005). *Compassion fatigue and the nurse.* Unpublished master's thesis, Nashville, Tennessee, Vanderbilt University.

Dunn, D. J. (2007, October). *A way of knowing, being, valuing and living with compassion energy: A unitary science perspective.* Paper presented at the Conference of the Rogerian Scholars, Cleveland, OH.

Dunn, D. J. (2009). The intentionality of compassion energy. *Holistic Nursing Practice 23*(4), 222-229.

Embee, L. (2006). *Reflective analysis.* Bucharest: Zeta Books.

Evans, M. (2005). On the job: Nurses reveal most, least enjoyable aspects of work. *Modern Health Care, 35*(14), 14-15.

Figley, C. (1995). *Compassion fatigue: Coping with secondary traumatic stress disorder in those who treat the traumatized.* New York: Brunner-Mazel.

Figley, C. (2002). Compassion fatigue: Psychotherapists' chronic lack of self-care. *Psychotherapy Practice 58,* 1433-1441.

Finfgeld-Connett, D. (2006). Meta-synthesis of caring in nursing. *Journal of Clinical Nursing, 17,* 196-204.

Fox, M. (1979). *A spirituality named compassion.* New York: HarperCollins.

Freudenberger, H. J. (1974). Staff burn-out. *Journal of Social Issues, 30*(1), 159-165.

Gadow, S. (1980). Existential advocacy. Philosophical foundations of nursing. In S. F. Spicker & S. Gadow (Eds), *Nursing: Images and ideals* (pp. 79-101). New York: Springer Publishing Company.

Gardiner, M., Sexton, R., Durbridge, M., & Garrard, K. (2005). The role of psychological well-being in retaining rural general practitioners. *Australian Journal of Rural Health, 13*(3), 149-155.

Gelinas, L., & Bohlen, C. (2002). The business case for retention. *Journal of Clinical Systems Management, 4*(7), 14-16.

Gelsema, T. I., van der Doef, M., Maes, S., Jansseen, M., Akerboom S., & Verhoven, C. (2006). A longitudinal study of job stress in the nursing profession: Causes and consequences. *Journal of Nursing Management, 14*(4), 289-299.

Gifford, B. D., Zammuto, R. F., & Goodman, E. A. (2002). The relationship between hospital unit culture and nurses' quality of work life. *Journal of Healthcare Management, 47*(1), 13-25.

Haalbesleben, J. R. B., & Buckley, M. R. (2004). Burnout in organizational life. *Journal of Management*, *30,* 859-879.

Haalbesleben, J. R. B., Wakefield, B. J., Wakefield D. S., & Cooper, L. B.. (2008). Nurse burnout and patient safety outcomes: Nurse safety perception versus reporting behavior. *Western Journal of Nursing Research, 30,* 560-577.

Halldorsdottir, S. (2007). A pyschoneuroimmunological view of the healing potential of professional caring in the face of human suffering. *International Journal for Human Caring, 11*(2), 32-39.

Hamilton, D. (1994). Constructing the mind of nursing. *Nursing History Review, 2,* 3-28.

Hart, S. (2005). Hospital ethical climates and registered nurses' turnover intentions. *Journal of Nursing Scholarship*, *37*(2), 173-177.

Hawkins, A. L., & Kratsch, L.S. (2004). Troubled units: Creating change. *Clinical Issues: Advanced Practice in Acute & Critical Care, 15*(2), 215-221.

Heidegger, M. (1962). *Being and time* (J. Macquarrie & E. Robinson, Trans.). New York: Harper & Row. (Original work published 1927)

Heidegger, M. (1977). *Basic writings.* New York: Harper Collins.

Henderson, V. (1961). *Basic principles of nursing care.* London: International Council of Nurses.

Hudacek, S. S. (2008). Dimensions of caring: A qualitative analysis of nurses' stories. *Journal of Nursing Education, 47*(3), 124-129.

Husserl, E. (1967). *Ideas: General introduction to pure phenomenology* (W. R. Boyce Gibson, Trans.). New York: Collier Books. (Original work published 1931)

Jackson, D., Clare, J., & Mannix, J. (2002). Who would want to be a nurse? Violence in the workplace-a factor in recruitment and retention. *Journal of Nursing Management, 10*(1), 13-20.

Jensen, K. P., Beck-Pettersson, S. R., & Segesten, K. M. (1993). The caring moment and the green thumb phenomenon among Swedish nurses. *Nursing Science Quarterly, 6*(2), 98-104.

Johns, C. (2005). With just a little bit of love: Reflection on dwelling with Kristen. *International Journal for Human Caring, 9*(1), 36-42.

Johnston, N. E. (2007). Meaning in suffering. In N. E. Johnston & A. Scholler-Jaquish, *Caring practice in the health professions* (pp. 7-59) Madison: University of Wisconsin Press.

Joinson, C. (1992). Compassion fatigue, *Nursing, 22,* 116-120.

Joint Commission on Accreditation of Healthcare Organizations. (2002). *Health care at the crossroads.* Retrieved December 14, 2008, from http://www.jcaho.org

Keidel, G. C. (2002). Burnout and compassion fatigue among hospice caregivers. *American Journal of Hospice and Palliative Care, 19*, 200-205.

Kelly, D., Ross, S. Gray, B., & Smith, P. (2000). Death, dying and emotional labor: Problematic dimensions of the bone marrow transplant nursing role. *Journal of Advanced Nursing, 32(*4), 952-960.

Koch, T. (1995). Interpretative approach in nursing research: The influences of Husserl and Heidegger. *Journal of Advanced Nursing, 21*, 827-836.

Kramer, M. (1974). *Reality shock: Why nurses leave nursing*, St. Louis: Mosby.

Larabee, J. H., Janney, M. A., Ostrow, C. L., Withrow, M. L., Hobbs, G. R., & Burant, C. (2003). Predicting registered nurse job satisfaction and intent to leave. *Journal of Nursing Administration, 33*(5) 271-283.

Latham, C. L., Hogan, M., & Ringl, K. (2008). Nurses supporting nurses: creating a mentoring program for staff nurses to improve the workforce environment. *Nursing Administration Quarterly, 32*(1), 27-39.

Lee, H., & Cummings, G. G. (2008). Factors influencing job satisfaction of front line nurse managers' systematic review. *Journal of Nursing Management, 16,* 768-783.

Lee, R. T., & Ashforth, B. E. (1996). A meta-analytic examination of correlates of three dimensions of burnout. *Journal of Applied Psychology, 81,* 123-133.

Leiter, M., & Laschinger, H. (2006). Relationships of work and practice environment to professional burnout: Testing a causal model. *Nursing research*, *55,* 137-146.

Lesniak, R. (2008). The lived experience of adolescent females who self-injure by cutting. *Dissertation Abstracts International, 69* (11). (AAT 3338723)

Lincoln, Y. S., & Guba, E. G. (1985). *Naturalistic inquiry,* Newbury Park, CA: Sage.

Locsin, R. (1998). Technologic competence as expression of caring in critical care settings. *Holistic Nursing Practice, 12*(4), 50-56.

Locsin, R. (2006). Technological competency as caring and the practice of knowing persons as whole. In M. E. Parker (Ed.), *Nursing theories & nursing practice* (2nd ed.; pp. 380-388). Philadelphia: F. A. Davis.

Lundberg, P. C., & Boonprasabhai, K. (2001). Meaning of good nursing care among Thai female last-year undergraduate nursing students. *Journal of Advanced Nursing, 34*(1), 35-42.

Luquette, J. (2007). Stress, compassion fatigue, and burnout: Effective self-care techniques for oncology. *Oncology Nursing Forum, 34*(2), 490.

Malinski, V. (2006). Martha E. Rogers' science of unitary human beings. In M. E. Parker (Ed.), *Nursing theories & nursing practice* (2nd ed.; pp. 160-166). Philadelphia: F. A. Davis.

Maslach, C. (1982). *Burnout: The cost of caring.* Englewood Cliffs, NJ: Prentice Hall.

McCann, L., & Pearlman, L. (1990). Vicarious traumatization: A framework for understanding the psychological effects of working with victims. *Journal of Traumamatic Stress, 3,* 131-149.

McCarthy, M. (1985). Burnout in psychiatric nursing. *Journal of Advanced Nursing, 10,* 305.

McMullen, L. (2007). Oncology nursing and compassion fatigue: Caring until it hurts. Who is caring for the caregiver? *Oncology Nursing Forum, 34*(2), 491-492.

Meadors, P., & Lamson, A. (2008). Compassion fatigue and secondary traumatization: Provider self care on intensive care units for children. *Journal of Pediatric Health,* 22(1), 24-34.

Merriam-Webster Online Dictionary. Retrieved June 4, 2008, from http://www.merriam-webster.com/dictionary/nurturance

Morse, J., Solberg, S, M., Neander, W. L., Bottoroff, J. L., & Johnson, J. L. (1990). Concepts of caring and caring as a concept. *Advances in Nursing Science, 13*(91), 1-14.

Mulcahy, C., & Betts, L. (2005). Transforming culture: An exploration of unit culture and nurse retention within a neonatal unit. *Journal of Nursing Management, 13*(6), 519-523.

Newman, M. A. (1994). *Health as expanding consciousness (*2nd ed.). New York: NLN.

Newman, M. A. (2008). *Transforming presence: The difference that nursing makes.* Philadelphia: F. A. Davis.

Nightingale, F. (1992). *Notes on nursing: What it is, and what it is not* (commemorative ed.). Philadelphia: Lippincott. (Original work published 1859)

O'Brien-Pallas, L., Duffield, C., & Alksnis, C. (2004). Who will be there to nurse? *Journal of Nursing Administration, 34*(6), 298-302.

Packer, M. J. (1989). Tracing the hermeneutic circle: Articulating an ontical study of moral conflicts. In M. J. Packer & R. B. Addison (Eds.), *Entering the circle: Hermeneutic investigation in psychology*, Albany: State University of New York Press.

Papadatou, D., Anagnostopoulos, F., & Monos, D. (1994). Factors contributing to the development of burnout in oncology nursing. *British Journal of Medical Psychology, 67,* 187-199.

Paterson, J. G., & Zderad, L. T. (1988). *Humanistic nursing.* New York: NLN.

Pearlman, L. (1998). Trauma and the self: A theoretical and clinical perspective. *Journal of Emotional Abuse, 1*, 7-25.

Peters, M. A. (2006). Compassion: An investigation into the experience of nursing faculty. *International Journal for Human Caring, 10*(3), 38-46.

Pharris, M. (2006). Margaret A. Newman's theory of health as expanding consciousness and its applications. In M. E. Parker (Ed.), *Nursing theories & nursing practice* (2nd ed.; pp. 217-234). Philadelphia: F. A. Davis.

Polkinghorne, D. (1983). *Methodology for the human sciences systems of inquiry.* Albany: State University New York Press.

Raup, G. H. (2008). The impact of ED nurse manager leadership style on staff nurse turnover and patient satisfaction in academic health center hospitals. *Journal of Emergency Nursing, 34*(5), 403-409.

Ray, M. A., & Turkel, M. C. (2002). The transformative process for nursing in workforce redevelopment. *Nursing Administration*, *26*(2), 1-14.

Roach, M. S. (2002). *Caring, the human mode of being: A blueprint for the health professions.* Ottawa: CHA Press.

Rogers, M. E. (1970). *An introduction to the theoretical basis of nursing.* Philadelphia: F. A. Davis.

Rose, J., & Glass, N. (2006). Community mental health nurses speak out: The critical relationship between emotional well-being and satisfying professional practice. *Collegian, 13*(4), 27.

Sabo, B. M. (2006). Compassion fatigue and nursing work: Can we accurately capture the consequences of caring work? *International Journal of Nursing Practice, 12*, 136-142.

Sabo, B. M. (2008). Adverse psychosocial consequences: compassion fatigue, burnout and vicarious traumatization: Are nurses who provide palliative and hematological cancer care vulnerable? *Indian Journal of Palliative Care,* 14(1), 23-29.

Salvage, J. (2006). Model thinking. *Nursing Standard, 20*(17), 24-25.

Sandowlowski, M. (1986). The problem of rigor in qualitative research. *Advances in Nursing Science, 8*(3), 27-37.

Sanghavi, D. M. (2006). What makes for a compassionate patient-caregiver relationship? *Joint Commission Journal on Quality and Patient Safety, 32*(5), 283-292.

Sappington, J. (2003). Nurturance: The spirit of holistic nursing. *Journal of Holistic Nursing, 21*(8), 8-19.

Schantz, M. L. (2007). Compassion: A concept analysis. *Nursing Forum, 42*(2), 48- 55.

Schein, E. (1999). Organizational cultures. *American Psychologist, 45,* 109-119.

Schwarz, T. (2005). Viewpoint. PTSD in nurses: On-the-job trauma may be driving nurses from the profession. *American Journal of Nursing, 105*(3), 13.

Sherwood, G. D. (1997a). Meta-synthesis of qualitative analyses of caring: Defining a therapeutic model of nursing. *Advanced Practice Nursing Quarterly, 3*(1), 32-42.

Sherwood, G. D. (1997b). Patterns of caring: The healing connection of interpersonal harmony. *International Journal for Human Caring, 1*(1), 30-38.

Simms, L. M., Erbin-Roesemann, M., Darga, A., & Coeling, H. (1990). Breaking the burnout barrier: resurrecting work excitement in nursing. *Nurse Economics, 8*(3), 177-187.

Sinclair, H., & Hamill, C. (2007). Does vicarious traumatization affect oncology nurses? A literature review. *European Journal of Oncology Nurses, 11,* 348-356.

Sirgo, C. E., & Coeling, H. (2005). Workgroup culture and the new graduate: Is this ICU right for you? *American Journal of Nursing, 105,* 85-87.

Smith, M. C. (1999). Caring and the science of unitary human beings. *Advances in Nursing Science, 21*(4), 14-28.

St. Pierre, C. (2006). What is so bad about feeling good? Student reflection on learning to care for self. *International Journal for Human Caring, 10*(2), 57.

Swanson, K. M. (1991). Empirical development of middle range theory of caring. *Nursing Research, 40,* 161-166.

Swenson, M. M., & Sims, S. L. (2007). Listening to learn: Narrative strategies and interpretive practices in clinical education. In N. L. Diekelmann, *Teaching the practitioners of care: New pedagogies for the health profession* (pp. 351-359). Madison: University of Wisconsin Press.

Todaro-Franceschi, V. (1999). The idea of energy as phenomenon and Rogerian science: Are they congruent? *Visions, 7*(1), 30-41.

U.S. Department of Health and Human Services. (2002). *Projected supply, demand and shortages of registered nurses: 2000-2020* Retrieved December 15, 2008, from http://www.ga.gov/new.iems/d01944.pdf

Valent, P. (2002). Diagnosis and treatment of helper stresses, traumas and illnesses. In C. Figley (Ed.), *Treating compassion fatigue* (pp. 17-37). New York: Brunner-Routledge.

van den Tooren, M., & de Jonge, J. (2008). Managing job stress in nursing: What kind of resources do we need? *Journal of Advanced Nursing, 63*(1), 75-84.

Watson, J. (1985). *Nursing: Human science and human care.* Norwalk, CT: Appleton-Century-Crofts.

Watson, J. (1999). *Postmodern nursing and beyond.* Edinburgh: Churchill Livingstone.

Watson, J. (2005). *Caring science as sacred science.* Philadelphia: F. A. Davis.

Watson, J. (2006). Jean Watson's theory of human caring. In M. E. Parker (Ed.), *Nursing theories & nursing practice* (2nd ed.; pp. 295-308). Philadelphia: F. A. Davis.

Watson, J., & Smith, M. C. (2001). Caring science and the science of unitary human beings: A trans-theoretical discourse for nursing knowledge development. *Journal of Advanced Nursing, 37*(5), 452-461.

Welch, M. (1999). Phenomenology and hermeneutics. In E. C. Polifroni & M. Welch, *Perspectives on philosophy of science in nursing: An historical and contemporary anthology* (pp. 235-246). Philadelphia: Lippincott.

Wilson, C. B., & Grams, K. (2007). Reflective journaling and self-care: The experience of MSN students in a course on caring. *International Journal for Human Caring, 11*(1), 16-21.

Woods, M. (1999). A nursing ethic: The moral voice of experienced nurses. *Nursing Ethics 6*(5), 423-433.

Younger, J. B. (1990). Literary works as a model of knowing. *Image: Journal of Nursing Scholarship, 22*(1), 39-43.

Zerwekh, J. (1993). Transcending life: The practice of wisdom of nursing hospice experts. *American Journal of Hospice and Palliative Care, 10*(5), 26-31.

www.ingramcontent.com/pod-product-compliance
Lightning Source LLC
LaVergne TN
LVHW011509220926
848485LV00016B/58
9781680534733